DIGITAL NEWS AND HIV CRIMINALIZATION

The Social Organization of Convergence Journalism

I0112479

For years, HIV activists and researchers have expressed deep concerns about the stigmatizing and sensational tone of news stories about HIV criminalization. *Digital News and HIV Criminalization* investigates the everyday work of journalists and uncovers how newswork routines are hooked into other institutions, including the criminal legal system, police, and public health, that regulate the daily lives of people living with HIV.

This lively institutional ethnography offers key insights into how the digital news media ecosystem is socially organized. It reveals that the fast-paced conditions of digital news media in the age of convergence journalism require the constant, rapid production of sensational news stories that will be consumed widely by online audiences, often resulting in news writing that perpetuates social harms connected to stigmatizing, racist, and anti-immigrant views. The book illustrates how biased reporting on HIV criminalization reflects broader trends in online news and presents opportunities for HIV activists to form coalitions with other groups negatively affected by the current landscape of convergence journalism.

Tracing how work that produces and circulates a standard genre of news story about HIV criminalization is coordinated across time and space, *Digital News and HIV Criminalization* offers a groundwork for political action aimed at disrupting the production of stigmatizing news stories.

COLIN HASTINGS is an assistant professor in the Department of Sociology and Legal Studies at the University of Waterloo.

Praise for *Digital News and HIV Criminalization*

"Colin Hastings's *Digital News and HIV Criminalization* meticulously details the symbiotic relationship between police and deadline-driven reporters, revealing how their interactions perpetuate stigmatizing narratives around HIV criminalization. Hastings's insightful analysis – part of an exciting new wave of activism-informed social science research from Canada – explores the strategic, astute efforts of advocates to challenge the supposed neutrality of mainstream news and law enforcement, advocating for a reclamation of the narrative space to support HIV justice."

Edwin J. Bernard, Executive Director,
HIV Justice Network

"Inspired by the groundbreaking writings of Dorothy E. Smith and George W. Smith, Colin Hastings has provided us with detailed descriptions of convergence journalists' work – their activities and the hurried conditions under which they labour – as it relates to criminalizing those with HIV. An excellent volume for scholars who are actively involved in their local communities, regardless of their areas of interest."

Paul Luken, Associate Professor Emeritus in Sociology,
University of West Georgia

"As an activist researcher, Colin Hastings unfolds for us how it happens that digital media journalists produce and circulate stories about HIV criminalization in the Canadian media, particularly versions that construct texts that are stigmatizing, objectifying, and alarmist. He skilfully examines journalists' work, organized by both tight deadlines and content ratings, in gathering sources across a wide array of institutional sites (criminal law, medical science, public health, digital information technology, and HIV advocacy) where the work practices of other people located elsewhere intersect and coordinate a journalist's newswork. In this respect, this book is one of only a few models that explores ruling relations across several institutional complexes in institutional ethnography (IE). Consequently, it is an important contribution to the expansive nature and often unexplored elements of Dorothy E. Smith's simple conceptualization of how we know the social through empirical inquiry and how IE inquiry can provide a map that social justice activists can use to make change."

Suzanne Vaughan, Associate Professor Emeritus of Sociology, Arizona State University

INSTITUTIONAL ETHNOGRAPHY: STUDIES IN THE SOCIAL ORGANIZATION OF KNOWLEDGE

Series Editor: Eric Mykhalovskiy

Institutional Ethnography: Studies in the Social Organization of Knowledge is a groundbreaking series that brings together prominent scholars from around the world who engage with institutional ethnography in a range of ways. Books in the series promote excellence and innovation in institutional ethnography inquiry while strengthening interdisciplinary dialogue between institutional ethnography and related forms of research. In a world being shaped by accelerated interconnection, this venue for exploring how ruling relations are created and operate, how they affect people's day-to-day lives, and how they can be transformed will make a lasting and meaningful impact on the field.

Digital News and HIV Criminalization

The Social Organization of Convergence Journalism

COLIN HASTINGS

UNIVERSITY OF TORONTO PRESS
Toronto Buffalo London

© University of Toronto Press 2024
Toronto Buffalo London
utorontopress.com
Printed in the USA

ISBN 978-1-4875-4464-5 (cloth)   ISBN 978-1-4875-4465-2 (EPUB)
ISBN 978-1-4875-5990-8 (paper)   ISBN 978-1-4875-4466-9 (PDF)

Institutional Ethnography: Studies in the Social Organization of Knowledge

---

Library and Archives Canada Cataloguing in Publication

Title: Digital news and HIV criminalization : the social organization of
   convergence journalism / Colin Hastings.
Names: Hastings, Colin (Assistant professor), author.
Description: Series statement: Institutional ethnography: studies in the
   social organization of knowledge | Includes bibliographical references
   and index.
Identifiers: Canadiana (print) 20240359305 | Canadiana (ebook) 20240359321 |
   ISBN 9781487544645 (hardcover) | ISBN 9781487559908 (softcover) |
   ISBN 9781487544669 (PDF) | ISBN 9781487544652 (EPUB)
Subjects: LCSH: HIV infections – Press coverage – Canada. |
   LCSH: AIDS (Disease) – Press coverage – Canada. | LCSH:
   Digital media – Social aspects – Canada. | LCSH: HIV positive
   persons – Legal status, laws, etc. – Canada.
Classification: LCC PN4914.A44 H37 2024 | DDC 070.4/496169792 – dc23

Cover design: Alexa Love
Cover image: iStock.com/The7Dew

We wish to acknowledge the land on which the University of Toronto Press
operates. This land is the traditional territory of the Wendat, the Anishnaabeg, the
Haudenosaunee, the Métis, and the Mississaugas of the Credit First Nation.

This book has been published with the help of a grant from the Federation for the
Humanities and Social Sciences, through the Awards to Scholarly Publications
Program, using funds provided by the Social Sciences and Humanities Research
Council of Canada.

University of Toronto Press acknowledges the financial support of the Government of
Canada, the Canada Council for the Arts, and the Ontario Arts Council, an agency of the
Government of Ontario, for its publishing activities.

Canada Council   Conseil des Arts
for the Arts   du Canada

ONTARIO ARTS COUNCIL
CONSEIL DES ARTS DE L'ONTARIO
an Ontario government agency
un organisme du gouvernement de l'Ontario

Funded by the   Financé par le
Government   gouvernement
of Canada   du Canada

Canada

Contents

Acknowledgments

This project has been a long journey, and I cannot imagine finishing it without the guidance and support I have received from generous mentors, colleagues, friends, and family along the way.

As a PhD student in the Department of Sociology at York University, I was lucky to work with a deeply insightful, inventive, and engaged dissertation committee: Eric Mykhalovskiy, Carmela Murdocca, and Lorna Weir. I am especially thankful to Eric for his endless encouragement and support. Eric generously introduced me to the sociologies, activist histories, activist organizations, and research networks that defined this project. I am hugely grateful for the ways that these all continue to shape my everyday work inside and outside the university.

I wrote this book in Montréal while doing a SSHRC Postdoctoral Fellowship in the Department of Sociology and Anthropology at Concordia University. Thank you to Martin French for making this ideal opportunity possible. This book, and my understanding of how to work in the university more broadly, have benefitted tremendously from Martin's wisdom and vision. Thank you to family and friends who make Montréal feel even more like a home, especially Mitch McLarnon, Alix Petter, and Finn McLarnon.

This project has been strengthened by conversations I have been fortunate to have with mentors and colleagues who intentionally cultivate supportive spaces for collective research and action. I am especially grateful for a number of conversations within the IE Division at SSSP over the years. I so appreciate the work that Dorothy Smith, Suzanne Vaughan, Paul Luken, Liza McCoy, Marjorie Devault, Janet Rankin, Naomi Nichols, Lauren Eastwood, and many others have done over decades to foster a generative and encouraging space for generations of institutional ethnographers. I am also incredibly thankful to learn from and organize alongside the brilliant people who have been part of the Canadian Coalition to Reform HIV Criminalization for the last number of years. Thank you especially to Alexander McClelland. Collaborations with Alex always bring out the best parts of getting to do this work.

A huge thank you to the University of Toronto Press for their support of this project. I am especially grateful to Jodi Lewchuk and the readers who reviewed the original manuscript and offered valuable feedback and suggestions that I believe made this book a much clearer and more useful text. I am grateful for Eric Mykhalovskiy's ongoing work to edit this series of institutional ethnographies with the University of Toronto Press and am eager to read the innovative works that are to come in this collection.

I made the final edits to this book from my new role in the Department of Sociology and Legal Studies at the University of Waterloo. I'm very grateful to the supportive colleagues in my department who have made the transition to my new position as gentle and as smooth as possible.

Overall, each stage of this journey has been made possible by an enduring circle of genuine, caring, kind, brilliant, and hilarious people who provide me with a steady homebase. Thanks and love especially to Mom and Dad, and Andrew and Lindsey, Annelies Cooper, Devin Clancy, June Cooper, Andrew Stokes, Craig Fortier, Daniel Wilson, Julia Gruson-Wood, Karl Gardner, Jeffery Ansloos, Patrick Byrne, Carey, Henry, and the Field of Dreamers Cooperative Softball Association. I'm very grateful.

DIGITAL NEWS AND HIV CRIMINALIZATION

Introduction

I believe I literally slept with the devil

HIV-positive immigrant ordered deported

HIV-infected man a danger, court told

The case of an AIDS-spreading lothario has ramifications for serial drunk drivers

Sex, lies, and AIDS: A young woman's summer romance has horrifying consequences

For years, these types of jarring headlines have introduced mass news media audiences to the issue of HIV criminalization. We can assume that news stories like these are often present in the everyday lives of news readers for mere moments. At the end of 2020, the average amount of time a user spent interacting with a piece of online content in North America was only 30.2 seconds. Such short bursts of attention are common in the contemporary digital news ecosystem, in which news and information are updated online constantly and travel faster than ever before (Castells 2009b; Usher 2018). Consuming news in this context has been likened to trying to drink out of a firehose (Jones 2020). However, when we pause to look closely at news about HIV criminalization we can gain important insights into how social knowledge about HIV is constructed. For example, when these types of headlines that demonize and objectify people living with HIV join the news cycle and flow onto our screens, they establish and re-establish damaging connections between HIV serostatus, crime, race, and migration status that have existed for decades and mediate the public's understandings of risk, safety, and health in meaningful ways.

There are important reasons to treat news discourse about HIV criminalization as an urgent social justice issue. First, these headlines start to show that mainstream news is a site where HIV stigma circulates. For as long as the virus has existed news media has spread stigmatizing, inaccurate, and alarmist information about HIV and AIDS. It is critical to recognize, however, that the social organization of knowledge about HIV in the press is not a social problem that is confined to the realm of journalism. As Gary Kinsman (2018, 312) writes, the social construction of knowledge about HIV is tied to the social organization "of stigmatization and discrimination along sexual, racializing, drug use and other lines; problems with the social organization of health care; problems with the for-profit capitalist organization of drug companies; and more." And so, in this book, studying how knowledge about HIV criminalization is constructed in the press means adding to a lineage of activist scholarship on the social relations of HIV that brings into view how HIV criminalization produces and is produced by broader social relations.

Another reason that it is crucial to delve into the social relations that generate these sorts of stigmatizing, objectifying, and alarmist headlines is because efforts to respond to and correct widespread stigmatizing misinformation about HIV have always been a key part of radical HIV activism. In Canada, one of the first stories that *The Body Politic* published about AIDS was titled "AIDS: Discounting the Promiscuity Theory," written by Bill Lewis in 1983 (ACT, n.d.). The article debunked the notion that HIV was spreading because "men were overloading their bodies with common sexually transmitted infections through multiple sexual encounters" and eroding their immune systems. Media and popular education work were also central to the early activities of *AIDS ACTION NOW!* Activists, including George Smith, organized a media committee and wrote columns for publications such as *AIDS ACTION NEWS!* and *Treatment Update* that helped circulate accurate and accessible information on the rights of people living with HIV, anonymous HIV testing, information on treatment and drug trials, and more that was not available in the mainstream press (AIDS Activist History Project, n.d.). For over thirty years, Black activists in particular have resisted racist media discourses that mobilize troubling links between race, morality, criminality, and HIV. For example, the spring issue of *Our Lives: Canada's First Black Women's Newspaper* includes a column authored by Carol Ann Allain (1988) entitled "AIDS Update: What Black Women Need to Know about AIDS" that critiques press coverage that centred on arguments about where AIDS started and "join[ed] in assigning blame for the disease rather than educating. But *AIDS is not a crime, it is a fatal disease*" (5; emphasis added).

Today, "HIV is not a crime" is a powerful refrain among HIV activists. The phrase commonly adorns stickers, T-shirts, and protest signs and is the name of an influential training academy that trains people living with HIV and activists on how to mobilize an end to HIV criminalization (SERO Project 2023). Since the first criminal charges related to HIV criminalization, a key aspect of activists' efforts to establish that "HIV is not a crime" has involved keeping track of what news media says about people living with HIV when covering criminal cases and intervening in the press to disrupt stigmatizing and objectifying discourses about people living with HIV. As the eye-catching headlines above start to show, news reports often instruct readers to conceptualize people who are accused of not disclosing their HIV-positive status to sex partners as morally culpable, dangerous criminals who are deserving of punishment. In this book I devote particular attention to ways the press fuels the criminalization of HIV in the early trajectory of reporting on a criminal non-disclosure case. Press coverage in the first stages of a criminal non-disclosure case often relies heavily on police news releases as sources and includes mugshot photos and other details of the case that derive from police. HIV advocates have expressed alarm about this type of reporting for decades. Not only is this genre of news deeply stigmatizing, these news reports also extend the work of police by calling on news readers to come forward as complainants or as people with additional information that police can use to build criminal charges against an individual living with HIV.

This book builds on a lineage of activism and scholarship about media representations of HIV criminalization by tracing duel, overlapping narratives. One arc of this project is a study of the social organization of knowledge about HIV criminalization. Research and activism related to news media representations of HIV often begin from the assumption that news texts do not simply portray the social world in a transparent or unfiltered way, but rather actively construct particular versions of reality. It is well documented that news media representations are most often crime genre stories that objectify people living with HIV and amplify stigma. This is particularly acute in news stories about people from BIPOC communities that circulate racist stereotypes that connect Black men with criminality and sexual violence. As the book outlines an empirical description of how a consistently racialized and stigmatizing genre of crime story about HIV criminalization is socially organized, one of the main goals is to illustrate that news texts are not simply the product of work that happens in the newsroom. The standard news discourse about HIV criminalization is made possible by work practices that are coordinated across different sites. This book shows that reporters link their newswork up to the work routines of their colleagues in the newsroom (such as technicians, editors, and other reporters) but also purposively hook their newswork up to others who work in different institutions (such as police and community-based HIV advocacy organizations). By tracing how work to produce and circulate a standard genre of news story about HIV criminalization is coordinated across time and space, this book aims to offer a groundwork for political action that tries to interrupt the production of stigmatizing news stories.

A close look at how news about HIV criminalization is produced offers a vantage point for examining the social organization of news more broadly. Thus, this book is also a study of how the broader contemporary news media ecosystem is put together. By applying institutional ethnographic research methods in newsrooms, I wanted to better understand how reporters organize their everyday newswork to keep step with the frantic pace of online news. The accounts that reporters, news editors, and web producers shared about producing news stories about HIV criminalization revealed that writing for digital news is premised mostly on work to activate online digital news texts (often emails, digital newswire texts, tweets, social media posts, online news articles from other news organizations, YouTube videos, etc.) and process them into news texts as fast and as often as possible. A main argument of this book is that this social organization of writing for digital news positions reporters to produce sensational news articles.

Objectives

Supporting Collective Efforts to End HIV Criminalization

Following the model put forth by George Smith (1990), I understand myself as an activist institutional ethnographer who seeks out ways of doing research that start from the local settings of my everyday work. Because this project is an exercise in extending the knowledge that I and fellow advocates have of the ruling relations of HIV criminalization, I want to situate myself in this research and advocacy work before moving forward.

I have been doing HIV advocacy work since 2010, when I worked as an education outreach coordinator at an AIDS service organization (ASO) in Ontario, Canada. When I left the ASO to start grad school in 2013, my departure coincided with an important development in the criminal-legal response to HIV in Canada. As I describe in further detail in the next chapter, in 2012 a landmark Supreme Court of Canada decision harshened the legal obligation to disclose one's HIV-positive status by introducing the concept of a "realistic possibility" of HIV transmission. What this means in practice is that people living with HIV in Canada are criminally charged for engaging in activities that, based on scientific evidence, pose a negligible HIV transmission risk, or in fact, no risk of transmitting HIV at all (Hastings et al. 2022).

There was a noticeable bifurcation in how the HIV sector responded to these changes in the criminal law. Many organizations such as AIDS ACTION NOW!, the Ontario Working Group on Criminal Law and HIV Exposure (CLHE), the Canadian HIV/AIDS Legal Network, the HIV/AIDS Legal Clinic of Ontario (HALCO), and others mobilized to challenge the use of the criminal law to respond to HIV non-disclosure. Other community-based organizations did not intend to address the socio-legal contexts in which people are required to disclose their HIV-positive status, but rather encouraged and supported people living with HIV to disclose their HIV-positive status to sexual partners and also to family, friends, and co-workers. These groups re-cast disclosure of one's HIV-positive status as an empowering and even gratifying practice. I started to study the social organization of HIV criminalization because I was concerned that these types of individualizing HIV disclosure interventions may be producing a new ethics of how to disclose one's HIV-positive status, and because they may overlook the social worlds in which people living with HIV are expected, or required, to disclose (Hastings 2019).

As a graduate student, I sought ways of doing social science research that aligned with activist work I was doing with community-based organizations dedicated to mobilizing resistance to HIV criminalization. During this period, I came to especially appreciate the works of institutional ethnographers who relate to studies of social organization as a way to extend people's knowledge of how their everyday worlds are put together, with a view to supporting collective action for social transformation (McCoy 2006; G. Smith 1990). As a sociologist working in the area of HIV and the criminal law, it can be challenging to locate inroads to research that meaningfully connect with the actual work of HIV activist movements. At conferences and advocacy group meetings, I have seen how physicians and scientists directly apply scientific research evidence on HIV transmission in order to add to calls to limit criminal prosecutions and convictions for HIV non-disclosure (Barré-Sinoussi et al. 2018; Loutfy et al. 2014). At the same time, I have worked alongside lawyers and policy experts who intervene directly in Canadian court proceedings, support defence attorneys, hold meetings with provincial and federal government policymakers, and assist people living with HIV through frontline support work.

This project builds on a lineage of research and activism that treats the mainstream press as a site of struggle in the context of HIV criminalization. Recognizing that the press is part of the broad complex of social relations that produce and reproduce HIV criminalization means that intervening on news production processes can contribute to ongoing collective efforts to end HIV criminalization. There are many ways that the press fuels HIV criminalization. For one, studies have emphasized that the press propels racist stereotypes and instructs readers to connect Black men with criminality and sexual violence (Adam et al. 2014; Miller 2005; Mykhalovskiy et al. 2021b; Mykhalovskiy 2011). The negative effects of media coverage have also been noted in Canadian studies that explore the experiences that people living with HIV have of HIV criminalization. In these studies, people living with HIV and service providers reported feelings of heightened HIV stigma and expressed concerns that media discourses exaggerate the risk of HIV transmission and amplify public fears about people living with HIV (Adam et al. 2015, 2016; African and Caribbean Council on HIV/AIDS in Ontario 2013; Mykhalovskiy et al. 2016). News reports of HIV criminalization have also been noted for the way that they extend the harmful, stigmatizing effects of HIV criminalization. People living with HIV who have faced criminal charges report that being eternally "googleable" in news stories about their criminal charges renders them vulnerable to harassment and discrimination and has posed major obstacles when trying to meet fundamental needs, such as securing employment or housing (McClelland 2019a). By uncovering how these problematic news stories are produced in the first place, I hope to support activists' efforts to effectively disrupt, challenge, and transform how this issue is presented to the public.

This book is grounded in the immediate concerns of HIV activists engaged in struggles over how the meaning of HIV criminalization is produced and circulates in the mainstream press. However, this project also may be of broader practical use because it sheds light on aspects of digital news media that are often beyond the vantage point of activists' daily work. Activists equipped with a fuller understanding of the social organization of the digital news media ecosystem are better positioned to effectively intervene in stigmatizing and sensational news media discourse on a range of pressing social justice issues.

Making Sense of Relentless Online News

At the same time, I hope this work can help us to think about the social organization of digital news production more broadly. For many of us, reading online news is not a discrete activity that somehow occurs in isolation from the rest of our everyday routines. Digital news content seeps into a web search we conduct at work, appears amid the social media feed we're scrolling, greets us on our iPhone home screen, and is emmeshed within the many other digital spaces we inhabit every day. As I spoke with reporters, I noticed that the weight I regularly feel reading online news content was mirrored by the pressure that they felt to rapidly produce online news content. Many reporters I spoke with expressed dismay about the frantic pace, commercialization, and subsequent sensational character of contemporary digital news media. An institutional ethnographic project cannot un-do these social relations of contemporary news media production on its own. It can, however, offer ways for reporters to talk back to objectified forms of knowledge that coordinate and manage their everyday work. For readers who work as newsmakers, this book may expand understandings of how their daily work hooks into the broader social relations of convergence journalism in ways that may not be visible in the course of their daily newswork routines. A more vivid conception of how the digital news media ecosystem is put together can support initiatives that foster nuanced, in-depth, ethical reporting.

Around the time I started this project the term "headline stress disorder" began to circulate in health and wellness and self-help discourses to describe how unrelenting sensational news comes to bear on the psyche of news audiences (Ramsey 2018; Rodriguez-Cayro 2018; Stosny 2017). An emblematic article quotes a clinical psychologist who recognizes that "being tuned into the 24-hour news cycle may fuel a lot of negative feelings like anxiety, sadness, and hopelessness ... a real sense of being out of control" (Spector 2017). This growing recognition of readers' anxious attachment to news was before March 2020, when a global pandemic sent many of us into our homes to try and make sense of our new physically distant reality by wading through endless streams of news stories about epidemic curves, infection rates, hospitalization rates, and public health regulations and guidance.

This book is a study of news *production*, but I want to start by calling attention to ways that relentlessly fast news (and often bad news) comes to bear on audiences so as to emphasize the noise of online news. This commotion makes it challenging for newsmakers and audiences to produce and access dependable information. However, reliable information is particularly indispensable in the face of the crises we encounter. To think sociologically about these issues, and to live our everyday lives in these conditions, we require sound information upon which we can mobilize meaningful responses.

I invite readers to sit with this book as a sort of respite from the din of online news. Perhaps no medium diverges from the rapid pace of online news more drastically than academic writing. As I conducted years of fieldwork and slowly wrote and rewrote this text, I was completely awestruck by the reporters I met who manage to produce multiple tightly written, publishable articles on an everyday basis. At the same time, I have appreciated how researching and writing this book has offered time and space to carefully reflect on how news production is organized to generate the content that arrives on our screens. I hope that reading this book also provides a vantage point for pausing and contemplating how we come to know about our social worlds.

Conceptual Framework

The consistently troubling patterns of news coverage of HIV criminal-ization invite sociological research that investigates how knowledge production about HIV criminalization is coordinated across various institutions and identifies how HIV advocates can interrupt the produc-tion of sensational and stigmatizing news media messages. I approach this work as a study in the social organization of knowledge and con-nect my analysis to studies of the medico-legal borderland.

Institutional Ethnography and Studies in the Social Organization of Knowledge

It is likely that many readers will arrive at this work by way of their interest, experience, or expertise in institutional ethnography (IE). As this book traces dual narratives that have to do with the social organi-zation of knowledge about HIV criminalization and the broader con-temporary news media ecosystem, it also works through the types of discussions that we often seem to have when we gather as institutional ethnographers at conferences and workshops or over videos calls and extended email chains. Discussions spurred by questions such as: What makes IE a distinct approach to sociology? What is IE's radical critique of sociology? What is its relationship to social theory? How does IE relate to other sociologies? And how can we apply IE in ways that con-tribute meaningfully to activist projects?

More immediately, this book also reflects on the more basic question of how one knows that an IE *is* an IE in the first place. Over the years I have often referred to my analytic approach using the term "studies in the social organization of knowledge" (SSOK) (Weir and Mykhalovskiy 2010, 23). I've sometimes leaned towards the label of SSOK rather than IE because of a concern that my work was not fully "IE enough." Rather than fret about the extent to which my research fits within the sometimes-rigid boundaries of IE's methodological exactitude, whether I was doing IE the "right way" or if my work sufficiently resembled what are routinely treated as exemplars of IE research, it was more comfortable to describe my work as "broadly inspired by Dorothy Smith's approach to empirical research" (Mykhalovskiy et al. 2021a, 54). I would often introduce a project using phrases such as "this work follows studies in the social organization of knowledge, a term used to refer to empirical research inspired by the work of Canadian feminist, Marxist scholar Dorothy Smith that takes 'ruling relations' as its object of study." The term "SSOK" seemed to communicate a commitment to the central features of IE while jettisoning formulations of IE as an inflexible, perhaps even formulaic, sociology.

In recent years I've been inspired by the works of institutional ethnographers who are pushing IE into exciting new directions. I've been especially motivated by projects that move IE into new empirical spaces, blend IE with other sociologies in creative ways, and apply IE to address pressing social justice issues. These works are important for the way that they remain deeply committed to the core of Smith's materialist social ontology while also inviting institutional ethnographers to imagine new possibilities for the sites and scopes of IEs. This is the lineage of IE I hope to contribute to in this book, and it is in conversations with these types of works that I feel most comfortable referring to the present project as an IE.

In the end, whether one employs the term SSOK or IE, there are core features of Dorothy Smith's (1987, 165; 2005, 151–2) approach to a sociology for people that we would want to adhere to closely. This includes resisting the tendency to begin sociological inquiry in social science discourse. The alternative to beginning in discourse is to start from the material standpoint of people's actual everyday work as they experience their everyday worlds. To support with maintaining an analytic focus on what people *do* in the course of their everyday lives, institutional ethnographers employ a broad and generous notion of the term "work." As Smith explains, in IE "work" extends "to anything done by people that takes time and effort, that they mean to do, that is done under definite conditions and with whatever means and tools, and they have to think about. It means much more than what is done on the job."

As institutional ethnographers see, hear, and understand what people *do* during their everyday lives they learn how the work people are doing in given local settings is coordinated with work other people are doing at different times and in different places (Mykhalovskiy et al. 2021a, 47). Within IE, this type of widespread coordination of everyday activities is referred to as "ruling relations" – the object of institutional ethnographic study. By ruling relations, Smith (1990, 14) is referring to the forms of ruling that are common in contemporary capitalist society, what she calls, "the total complex of activities by which our kind of society is managed and administrated." Sociologists who adopt Smith's approach to empirically studying the social organization of ruling relations have mostly called attention to the ways that people's work activities are coordinated *within* professional, formal, managerial settings, such as health care, education, and the social service sector. A unique contribution of the present project is that it applies an institutional ethnographic lens to study the everyday work people do outside of managerial settings and is especially interested how people's work is coordinated *across* disparate sites.

As is typical for an IE project, this study did not start in sociological literature but was propelled by a need to understand what activists are up against and how the conditions that they are confronting are held in place. In a context in which HIV activists label news media content about HIV criminalization as a source of profoundly stigmatizing discourse and work to mobilize counter discourses, IE offers a way to learn about the broad coordinated activities that people actually do to produce problematic news stories in the first place. During conversations with reporters, I learned about various routine work practices that comprise newswork. These work activities include researching and identifying a newsworthy story, pitching news stories to editors, identifying sources for interviews, conducting interviews, and writing and editing work to move the news article into print and online publications. Recognizing how these various newswork activities are coordinated across a news organization tells us something about the ruling relations of news media, but it does not tell us the whole story of how news articles about HIV criminalization happen.

This research began in newsrooms talking with reporters about their everyday work; however, my analytic attention was not limited to the newsroom or the functional complex of news media. As reporters described their routine work it became clear that the news stories they wrote would not be possible without the work that others do within other functional complexes. For example, the work that a reporter does to write a news story about HIV criminalization relies on the work that police communications departments do to produce press releases about people who have been criminally charged in cases of HIV non-disclosure and the work that community-based HIV advocacy organizations do to intervene in stigmatizing news stories and produce counter discourses. Thus, while my study started with a series of interviews in newsrooms, I eventually found myself travelling to police stations and community-based HIV organizations to conduct interviews with people about the work they do there. Using institutional ethnographic approaches to collecting and analysing people's accounts of their work practices in this range of settings makes it possible to show the broadly coordinated activities that produce (and also work to disrupt) a standard genre of news story about HIV criminalization.

Extending this IE beyond its original site of the newsroom and investigating how work activities are coordinated across disparate sites responds to what Eric Mykhalovskiy and I have referred to in other works as "the single institution tendency" in IE (Hastings and Mykhalovskiy 2023). We use the phrase to describe a trend in some institutional ethnographic research to focus on a single institution (e.g., health care, education, policing, or social services) rather than on how institutional practices intersect across functional complexes. Our concern is that the single institution tendency restricts the potential of institutional ethnographic analyses of relations that are not neatly packaged, bounded, or contained as people experience them in their everyday lives (McCoy 2006). Using institutional ethnographic methods to illuminate how news content is produced through the broad concerting of work practices can yield a broader perspective on how news about HIV criminalization is accomplished.

With this sense of IE in mind, one way to demonstrate IE's distinct approach is to consider different ways that a sociologist could design a study of news media reports of HIV criminalization. For instance, one could begin research into news media discourse of HIV criminalization in sociological literature. Such an approach might centre on applying or testing theoretical concepts from social constructionist studies of how media produce images of crime and justice. In social constructionist approaches to media studies, research examines "social competition among different constructions of reality over being accepted as the general, dominant construction of reality" (Surette 1998, 8). Researchers are interested in understanding how the media interprets and distributes what becomes society's generally accepted view. A study of news discourse of HIV criminalization that adopted a social constructionist approach would be committed to identifying and categorizing the key "claims" that are made about HIV criminalization in the press; recognizing the "claim-makers" who put forward these claims; understanding the way that some "claim-makers" come to "own the issue" in the press; and acknowledging "linkages" between HIV criminalization and other issues in the news (9–10). This approach positions the sociologist to produce a theory about the role of mass media in constructing shared meanings (6).

IE studies of social relations take a different approach. Rather than collecting data that can be used to test or produce a theory about news media representation of HIV criminalization, a central goal of this book is to identify how people's work practices in disparate sites are coordinated over time and space to make the standard news discourse about HIV criminalization possible. As Campbell and Gregor (2008, 89–90) describe:

> Where ethnographers in the conventional mode conduct tests (for example, triangulation) to give evidential weight to specific views, the institutional ethnographer attempts to explicate how the local settings, including local understandings and explanations, are brought into being – so that informants can talk about their experiences in the way they do ... getting to an account that explicates the social relations of the setting is what an institutional ethnographic account is about.

In order to produce analytic descriptions of social relations, institutional ethnographers read interview transcripts for social organization, seeking to uncover how people's activities are coordinated trans-locally. The analytic practice of reading for social organization rests on the assumption that social organization is built into people's way of speaking, that we can "find in their talk particular moments of participation in social relations that hook their local experience to the work of others elsewhere, known, and unknown" (D.E. Smith 2002, 31). As I read interview transcripts, I was alert for how peoples' accounts of their work connect them to the work that others are doing in other social sites. For example, this meant looking closely for moments in reporters' accounts of their newswork where they described how they used a text (such as a representation of a statistic that quantifies web traffic [the number of times a news article they wrote is "clicked," "liked," or "shared"], a tweet, or a police report) that arrived at their work site from elsewhere in a way that made it possible for them to produce a news report.

As we will see in the next chapter, the everyday newswork of reporters and HIV activists who shape news content about HIV criminalization have not been widely recognized as part of the broader ruling relations that produce and sustain HIV criminalization in Canada. However, bringing these activities into view reveals that HIV criminalization partly occurs through journalistic work practices that produce news texts that enable the social relations of HIV criminalization in Canada to exist extra-locally and to coordinate multiple local sites of people's everyday activities (D.E. Smith 2001, 174). In so doing, the book enhances understandings of how HIV criminalization works, how it's put together (Weir and Mykhalovskiy 2010, 24).

Thinking Sociologically about the Medico-Legal Borderland

My institutional ethnographic approach to studying intersecting social relations is bolstered by the work of scholars who have located their studies of HIV criminalization in an analytical and empirical space called "the medico-legal borderland" (McClelland 2013; Sanders 2014). The "medico-legal borderland" is a concept used to denote sites in which health care and criminal-legal practices overlap (Timmermans and Gabe 2002). It is a useful sociological concept for researchers conducting empirical studies of the social processes and social effects of HIV criminalization because it prompts researchers to consider the particular forms of overlapping social control and hybrid health/crime subjects that emerge when criminal law and health care governance converge (Mykhalovskiy 2011, 674).

Studies of HIV criminalization that are attuned to the medico-legal borderland are significant because they push past what has been called the "criminal law–person living with HIV dyad" (Mykhalovskiy 2011). The "criminal law–person living with HIV dyad" denotes a common feature of empirically based, social science research on the public health implications of HIV criminalization in which attention is fixed on the activities of people living with HIV and populations who are understood to be "at-risk" of contracting HIV (Dodds and Keogh 2006; Galletly and Dickson-Gomez 2009). For example, social scientists with an interest in HIV criminalization have focused on the ways that people living with HIV understand criminal legal obligations to disclose one's HIV status, and the relationship between one's sexual risk behaviour and the presence of laws that govern disclosure (Burris et al. 2007; Dodds, Bourne, and Weait 2009). This line of research on the public health impact of HIV criminalization that concentrates on the activities of people living with HIV has been useful for confirming that criminal laws do not enhance activities that prevent HIV transmission and cautioning against the use of the criminal law as a response to HIV. This book builds on research that concentrates on the activities of people living with HIV by highlighting a wider range of actors whose activities are also shaped by the social relations that HIV criminalization organizes.

In recent years, sociologists studying HIV criminalization have extended studies of the medico-legal borderland by showing how HIV criminalization is produced and reproduced through work practices that are coordinated across institutions. For instance, Alexander McClelland (2019a) examines how people living with HIV come to be known, defined, classified, and understood as risks and criminals through diverse forms of authoritative and expert knowledge. His work illustrates how HIV criminalization is accomplished through intertwining processes of various institutions, including public health, the criminal legal system, corrections institutions, policing, civil society groups, and community-based organizations.

Likewise, Chris Sanders's (2015) study of how the realms of criminal law and public health merge directs attention to ways that the criminal law organizes the reasoning and documentary practices of public health nurses; Catherine Dodds and colleagues (2015) illustrate how prosecutions for HIV transmission influence, and in some cases disrupt, the way that health care providers deliver HIV services; and Martin French (2015) calls attention to ways that the criminal-legal regulation of HIV non-disclosure comes to bear on public health service providers who offer post-test HIV counselling. Each of these sociologists productively shifts perspectives on HIV criminalization beyond the "criminal law-PHA behaviour dyad" to bring into view the complex of professional and community work practices that are affected by the intersecting health care and criminal-legal governance of HIV non-disclosure. In so doing, they contribute to a more relational understanding of HIV criminalization than is possible when attention remains fixed solely on the way that people living with HIV navigate the criminal-legal obligation to disclose one's HIV-positive status prior to sex. This book is informed by the work of sociologists who locate their inquiries into the criminalization of HIV non-disclosure in the analytical and empirical space of the medico-legal borderland and understand HIV criminalization as a complex of activities that involves a range of actors. Yet my analysis takes a different approach. I do not investigate how criminalization affects the counselling or other activities of health care professionals or those involved in efforts to prevent HIV transmission. Instead, my study starts by exploring how HIV criminalization shapes the work practices of news reporters who in turn inform public knowledge of HIV criminalization.

Chapter Overview

My study of how the social relations of HIV criminalization traverse the realms of news media, police, and community-based HIV advocacy organizations develops in four remaining chapters. In the next chapter, I provide a deeper description of the criminal law governance of HIV non-disclosure in Canada and trace recent changes in the ways this law has been applied. I outline some of activists' main concerns about how HIV criminalization has been portrayed in the mainstream Canadian press and describe key trends and patterns in news coverage based on critical discourse analyses of news articles. In the next chapter I also explain the context of convergence journalism in Canada and describe some of the major changes that digital news ecosystems have undergone in recent years. I argue that the social organization of reporters' work in the context of convergence journalism makes it exceedingly difficult for reporters to interrupt the longstanding trend of stigmatizing and objectifying news discourse about HIV criminalization.

Chapter 2 is the first of three chapters based on my institutional ethnographic fieldwork.[1] I draw on interviews with reporters to examine the everyday work that they do to produce digital news content. Reporters' accounts of their newswork in this chapter illustrate that they are under tremendous pressure to produce a seemingly unending stream of digital news content that will be widely consumed online. This chapter extends sociological studies of new production by showing that to keep pace with the unrelenting demands of convergence journalism, reporters' work centres largely on repurposing and distributing digital source texts – a newswork practice I call "writing for digital news." My main argument in this chapter is that writing for digital news makes it likely that news accounts of HIV criminalization will continue to be written as sensational crime genre stories.

My analysis in chapter 3 concentrates specifically on the ways that reporters' newswork connects to corporate communications departments within police forces, because journalists I interviewed consistently named police news releases as their most significant source of news stories about HIV criminal non-disclosure cases. I argue that as reporters strategically select segments of text from police news releases

---

1 See the appendix for detailed descriptions of research method.

and recontextualize it as news, they facilitate the flow of police knowledge and reasoning into the mainstream press. This section of the book extends sociological studies of the "police mission drift" by showing that the coordination of police communications work and reporters' newswork is an integral aspect of the social organization of knowledge about HIV criminalization.

In chapter 4, I turn my attention to the work of community-based HIV advocates who endeavour to interrupt crime genre reporting about HIV criminalization. I draw on advocates' descriptions of their media activities to bring forward three types of media intervention work: work as spokespeople on the issue of HIV criminalization in the press, work to produce media texts, and work to cultivate relationships with reporters. I argue that advocates' interactions with the press are more than simply encounters between representatives of community organizations and a representative of a news organization. Reading advocates' accounts of their media work for social organization shows that their interactions with the press are highly strategic initiatives to coordinate diverse knowledge and expertise of HIV advocates and align them with the relevancies of reporters.

The book concludes in chapter 5 by recapping key findings and themes, and recommending next steps for advocacy and research on HIV criminalization, health news, and the mainstream press. I also offer thoughts on what the production of news about HIV criminalization tells us about the circulation of news media information about present public health crises and how these lessons may equip us to navigate the "infodemic" that comes with COVID-19.

Chapter One

HIV Criminalization, Activism, and News Media in Canada

Before we meet journalists and HIV activists who shape news content about HIV criminalization, it's helpful to step back and consider the contexts and conditions in which they work. This chapter helps us to start to acknowledge how news media reproduce the social relations of HIV criminalization and also how the work of journalists is hooked into the work people do across disparate settings, including criminal law, medical science, public health, HIV advocacy, and digital information technology. While this chapter is organized in a way that treats these realms as discrete categories, the accounts of people I speak with in the following chapters illustrate how these institutions often blend into and overlap with each other.

HIV Criminalization

HIV criminalization is a global phenomenon and a major concern of HIV activists around the world. While the term can mean different things across jurisdictions, broadly, it refers to "the unjust application of criminal law to people living with HIV for nonmalicious HIV transmission, perceived or potential HIV exposure, or non-disclosure of known HIV-positive status" (Bernard, Symington, and Beaumont 2022, S395). The HIV Justice Network's monitoring and analysis of HIV-related criminal laws indicates that 130 countries have unjustly criminalized people living with HIV over the course of the epidemic.

The criminal law is applied to alleged instances of HIV exposure, transmission, or non-disclosure of one's HIV-positive status in different ways around the world. While some jurisdictions apply HIV-specific statutes, others apply a wide range of general criminal laws (for example, sexual assault, bodily harm, attempted murder) (Bernard, Symington, and Beaumont 2022, S395). In the Canadian context, non-disclosure of HIV status has been criminalized under general criminal laws since the first case in 1989, most often as aggravated sexual assault. The application of general criminal laws to HIV cases in Canada has led to Canada becoming a global hotspot for HIV criminalization (HIV Justice Network 2023).

HIV non-disclosure has been consistently prosecuted under sexual assault laws in Canada since the 1998 Supreme Court ruling in *R. v. Cuerrier*. In 1998, the Supreme Court of Canada (SCC) established that non-disclosure of one's HIV status may amount to fraud vitiating consent to sex in some circumstances under paragraph 265 (3) (c) of the Criminal Code. Specifically, the court ruled that people living with HIV have a legal obligation to disclose their HIV-positive status to sexual partners before sex that poses a "significant risk" of HIV transmission. The legal duty to disclose one's HIV-positive status intensified in 2012 as the SCC ruled that there is a legal requirement to disclose one's HIV-positive status before having sex that poses a "realistic possibility" of HIV transmission. In its decision, the court stated that "as a general matter, a realistic possibility of transmission of HIV is negated if (i) the accused's viral load at the time of sexual relations was low and (ii) condom protection was used" (SCC 47 at para. 94).

One of the common criticisms of HIV criminalization around the world is that the criminal law is applied in extremely broad ways. The HIV Justice Network is aware of 50 countries that actively prosecute people living with HIV for sexual acts that may or may not actually risk HIV transmission (HIV Justice Network 2023). This problem of "over criminalization" is a defining feature of HIV criminalization in Canada as well (Housfather 2019). A main critique of the 2012 SCC decision is that a "realistic possibility" of HIV transmission can include activities that, based on current scientific evidence, pose a negligible HIV transmission risk, or no risk of HIV transmission at all. In fact, most Canadian prosecutions have been for cases that did not involve HIV transmission (Hastings et al. 2022). In Canada, a person living with HIV can go to prison and be registered as a sex offender for life for not disclosing their HIV-positive status – regardless of whether transmission occurred or was even a realistic possibility. The exceptionally punitive character of HIV criminalization in Canada is also evident in trends that suggest that HIV non-disclosure cases have very high rates of conviction and that a large proportion of cases result in prison sentences.

Another consistent critique of HIV criminalization globally centres on the discriminatory nature of these laws. Analysis of global trends in prosecutions related to HIV criminalization suggest "HIV criminalization serves as a proxy for discrimination based on class, ethnicity, gender identity, migrant status, race, sex, sexual orientation, and other markers of social vulnerability" (Bernard, Symington, and Beaumont 2022, S395). These trends hold true in Canada where there is evidence that the criminal law comes to bear in particularly harsh ways on people living with HIV who are marginalized by structural conditions. Like many aspects of a criminal legal system rooted in settler colonialism, Canadian criminal law is applied in discriminatory ways in the context of HIV criminalization. Recent data shows that "when Black and Indigenous people face HIV criminalization charges they are convicted at a higher rate, acquitted at a lower rate, and are more likely to face prison sentences compared to white people who face similar charges" (Hastings et al. 2022). Analysis of HIV criminalization in Canada also recognizes various ways that the broader effects of HIV criminalization are patterned by inequities related to gender and sexual orientation. The gendered character of HIV criminalization is shown when the criminal law is weaponized by a partner who threatens to accuse a sexual partner of failing to disclose their HIV status, or the ways in which women living with HIV report that HIV criminalization contributes to their being surveilled by other systems, such as child welfare (HIV Legal Network 2021). The harmful effects of HIV criminalization in Canada are of course exacerbated for those with precarious migration status who face potential deportation should they face criminal charges. Efforts to end HIV criminalization should be understood as part of a broader movement to resist discriminatory policing, surveillance, and criminal law practices.

Data on the ways that the criminal law is applied in cases of alleged HIV non-disclosure offers some insight into the injustices of HIV criminalization but doesn't tell the entire story about how criminalization comes to bear on people living with HIV. HIV criminalization not only happens in criminal courts, it also happens as people living with HIV go about their everyday lives under the constant threat of being criminalized and as they confront HIV stigma that has been reinforced in the mainstream press coverage of HIV criminal cases for years. Efforts to change how the news media writes about HIV criminalization may not directly contribute to ending HIV criminalization, but it can intervene in the production and circulation of messages that support such a use of the criminal law and mobilize discourses that counter standard crime genre accounts of the issue.

Activism to Resist and Reform HIV Criminalization in Canada

While there are myriad intersecting and overlapping harms associated with HIV criminalization, thanks to the sustained advocacy work of HIV activists around the world, many jurisdictions are currently repealing criminal laws used to prosecute HIV transmission, exposure, or non-disclosure or reforming laws to narrow their scope. Such a campaign is underway in Canada where communities of people who live with HIV and advocates have been mobilizing against HIV criminalization for more than 25 years. Since 2016 the movement has been largely coordinated and led by the Canadian Coalition to Reform HIV Criminalization (CCRHC) – a coalition of people, including those living with HIV, community organizations, lawyers, and researchers, who advocate for ways to limit and ultimately eradicate HIV criminalization in Canada (HIV Justice Network 2023). Thanks in large part to the sustained advocacy work of the Coalition there has been a series of promising developments at the federal level in recent years that have helped to narrow the scope of HIV criminalization in Canada.

First, on World AIDS Day 2016, the Federal Attorney General recognized HIV criminalization as a "problem of overcriminalization." On the same day a year later, Justice Canada released a report entitled "Criminal Justice System's Response to the Non-Disclosure of HIV," which includes significant recommendations to limit prosecutions against people living with HIV. In 2018, the Federal Attorney General drew on this report to publish a binding directive to the Public Prosecution Service of Canada that guided against prosecution in cases in which a person has a suppressed viral load, used condoms, engaged only in oral sex, or was taking treatment as prescribed. In June 2019, the House of Commons Standing Committee on Justice and Human Rights released a report that integrated several important recommendations from HIV advocates to further limit the broad, unscientific, and unjust use of the criminal law against people living with HIV. The most significant recommendations included calls to remove HIV non-disclosure from the reach of sexual assault law and to narrow the criminalization of HIV to actual transmission only (Housfather 2019, 15).

There was another major step towards criminal law reform in Canada in 2022 in the form of a federal government review and public consultation on HIV criminalization. The government's consultation invited stakeholders and the general public to respond to thirteen questions in an online survey to inform legislation that it may introduce in Parliament. Community-based organizations, such as the CCRHC, welcomed the consultation as an important move towards law reform and continue to meet with government ministers and their staffs to argue for federal reforms to limit HIV criminalization and to discuss how findings from this consultation may be translated into law.

As those who resist HIV criminalization in Canada intervene in court decisions, engage with political leaders and policymakers, provide public legal education, and draft policy alternatives with a view to producing policy changes, they also work to shape broader public opinion on this issue. The mainstream press is one of the main vehicles that advocates use to intervene in the court of public opinion. Most of my work with the CCRHC has been on the Coalition's media working group. The bulk of the working group's activities fall into one of two categories. One way we engage with the media is by mobilizing critiques about how mainstream media has covered HIV criminal cases. In Canada there is a long lineage of people living with HIV, many AIDS service organizations (ASOs), HIV activist collectives, legal organizations, and researchers who have expressed deep concerns about how HIV criminalization is portrayed in the mainstream press and worked to intervene in media coverage. African, Caribbean, and Black communities have been leaders in mobilizing concerns about how problematic forms of racist and anti-migrant discourse intersect in news coverage of HIV criminalization. A key statement of those concerns is a report produced by the African and Caribbean Council on HIV/AIDS in Ontario (Mykhalovskiy et al. 2016). The report documents well-founded concerns that "media coverage of these cases will increase the stigma against our communities as Black people living with HIV are inaccurately portrayed as irresponsible sexual predators, infecting 'innocent Canadians'" (African and Caribbean Council on HIV/AIDS in Ontario 2013, 10). The report also describes the way that reporters "focus unnecessarily on the accused person's race, ethnicity and immigration status ... [and] lead the public to think that Black people are criminally inclined. They create fear and hostility toward ACB people generally ... Just as the law must change, so too must the stories' portrayal in the media" (14).

To reinforce community concerns about racialization and anti-migrant discourses in newspaper coverage of HIV criminalization, community-based HIV advocates have connected with researchers who have conducted quantitative and qualitative studies of the corpus of newspaper articles about HIV criminalization in Canada. For example, colleagues and I have published research findings that underline widespread concern about the way that Black men (especially those who came to Canada as migrants and refugees) are dramatically overrepresented in newspaper coverage of HIV non-disclosure criminal cases.

African, Caribbean, and Black men who are living with HIV and come to Canada as migrants or refugees "are featured in newspaper articles four times more often than would be expected on the basis of the proportion of all defendants involved in criminal cases that they account for" (Mykhalovskiy et al. 2016, 53). Our research also confirms that news coverage of HIV criminalization relies on racialized tropes that negatively characterize Black men as threats to individual "victims" and to the imagined white settler Canadian nation (Hastings et al. 2020; Mykhalovskiy et al. 2021b). This type of data has been useful for calling attention to the problematic and skewed character of news reports of HIV criminalization in diverse spaces, such as HIV community meetings, research conferences, and within the mainstream press (Easton 2016; Goh 2017; Keung 2016).

This book looks closely at how such a deeply stigmatizing news discourse about HIV criminalization is produced because for years this genre defined mainstream coverage of the issue and was a major concern among people living with HIV and those working in the movement to end HIV criminalization. Thanks in large part to the efforts of advocates there have been fewer criminal charges and convictions related to HIV non-disclosure in recent years, and in turn, fewer news stories reporting on criminal cases. Much of the media work of the CCRHC now focuses on mobilizing critiques about HIV criminalization in the press and shoring up public support for law reform. This type of intervention is largely premised on the work that HIV activists do as spokespeople to translate complex legal arguments and medical science on HIV transmission to mass audiences. Recently, HIV advocates have successfully moved critiques that, for the most part, tend to circulate in alternative presses, activist publications, and within HIV organizations, into the mainstream press. For example, advocates' calls to enact consistent policies to limit HIV non-disclosure prosecutions were recently the topic of articles in the *Globe and Mail* and the *Toronto Star* (Bains 2019; Emmanuel 2019; Gallant 2019; Wilson 2022). As advocates continue the push to end HIV criminalization and change the way that HIV criminalization is talked about, my hope is that this study can contribute to strategies for engaging with the mainstream press on this complex issue.

Media Representations, Stigma, and HIV Criminalization

Since the mid-1980s, social scientists have taken media representations of HIV seriously. Many have argued that mass media misrepresents those affected by HIV, and in so doing, fuels moral panic about the virus (Albert 1986; Baker 1986; Bayer 1991; Gillett 2003; Lester 1992; D. Miller and Williams 1993; Naylor 1985; Sontag 1989; Watney 1987). The first studies of mass media representations of HIV often focused on how the press conveyed moralizing messages about "deviant" gay men – spurring homophobia and broader AIDS phobia (Lupton 1994; Patton 1986). More recent studies of media representations of HIV have shown that the press continues to spread misinformation and reinforce anxieties about HIV by representing particular groups of people living with HIV, especially Black, Indigenous, and people of colour, people who have recently migrated, people who sell sex, and people who use drugs as "dangerous others" (Lupton 1999; McKay et al. 2011; Persson and Newman 2008).

In recent years, studies of news media and HIV have accentuated the particularly problematic ways that news media produce meanings of HIV criminalization. Research shows that news media reports of HIV criminal non-disclosure cases are commonly reductionist accounts that diminish complex cases to descriptions of sharp criminal–victim dichotomies (Petty 2005; Weait 2007). Scholarly critiques of media reports of criminalization also illuminate that media rely on sensational language, reproduce negative stereotypes of offenders, and exaggerate the threat that people living with HIV pose to the general public (Flavin 2000; Patton 2005). A distinguishing feature of news reports of HIV criminalization is that they objectify people living with HIV as morally blameworthy criminals. This trend has shown to be especially pronounced when criminal cases related to HIV disclosure involve people who are Black, Indigenous, and people of colour and people who arrived in jurisdictions as migrants or refugees (Bird and Dardenne 2009; McKay et al. 2011; J. Miller 2005; Mykhalovskiy et al. 2021b; Persson and Newman 2008). In the Canadian context, June Callwood's 1995 book *Trial without End: A Shocking Story of Women and AIDS* arguably set the scene for much of what followed in Canadian reporting on HIV criminalization. As Jennifer Kilty (2021, 342) writes, Callwood's narrative "shores up support for the problematic construction of Black and African immigrant men as inherently duplicitous threats to the sexual health and safety of Canadian women and thus for the punitive governmentalities (vengeance, anger, retribution) that underlie HIV criminalization efforts."

News reports that objectify people living with HIV as criminal subjects and produce defendants as morally reprehensible and blameworthy are not unique to people of colour or those who have come to Canada as migrants or refugees. For example, a close look at the media coverage of a white Canadian woman who has faced criminal

HIV non-disclosure charges shows that news stories are consistently premised on a criminal–victim dichotomy, hyper-sexual representations of the person facing charges, and the exaggeration of the risk of HIV transmission that she poses (Kilty and Bogosavljevic 2019; Roth and Sanders 2018). However, it is especially important to call attention to ways that these types of objectifying discourses are often paired with and amplify strategies that produce racial difference in news stories about HIV criminalization.

This line of social science research that emphasizes problematic media messages about HIV can be understood as part of broader sociological discussions of HIV stigma. Typically, research on HIV stigma takes Erving Goffman's classic work as its point of departure. Goffman defines stigma as "'an attribute that is significantly discrediting' which, in the eye of society, serves to reduce the person who possesses it" (Goffman 1963; Parker and Aggleton 2003, 14). This conception of stigma, write Richard Parker and Peter Aggleton, tends to consider HIV- and AIDS-related stigma in highly emotional terms. They point out that the analytic focus of studies of HIV stigma often remain fixed on stigma as "anger and other negative feelings towards people living with HIV … or 'stigmatizing attitudes' that are correlated with misunderstandings and misinformation concerning the modes of HIV transmission" (15).

I want to place this book in line with the work of Parker and Aggleton (2003, 19), who encourage a move beyond conceptions of HIV stigma "as a thing which individuals pose on others." Instead, I understand HIV stigmatization "as a process linked to competition for power and the legitimization of social hierarchy and inequality." As Parker and Aggleton write,

> It is important to better understand how stigma is used by individuals, communities and the state to produce and reproduce social inequality. It is also important to recognize how understanding of stigma and discrimination in these terms encourages a focus on the political economy of stigmatization and its links to social exclusion. (17)

This IE of media production intends to enhance understandings of stigmatization as a process that is tied to the reproduction of inequitable power relations. While previous studies make clear that the content of media messages about HIV convey negative attitudes about people living with HIV and spread misinformation, researchers have yet to empirically investigate how these media messages about HIV are produced in the first place. To correct for that gap, this study empirically investigates how the work of journalists is connected to work in other institutions that produce and reproduce power and control over people living with HIV – such as the criminal justice system, police, and public health.

Studies of Digital Newsmaking

This book adds to a lineage of newsroom ethnographies that dates back to the 1950s. There is a sense among some media researchers that the "golden period of media production studies" has passed (Tumber 1999, xvi). Yet other news media researchers, such as Chris Paterson (2008), encourage ethnographers to return to the newsroom. He cautions that the shift away from ethnographic studies of news production was "unfortunate and premature" because ethnographic analyses of newsrooms offer a unique and valuable perspective on the actual spaces where decisions related to genres, routines, values, and news products are made (3). Indeed, by venturing into newsrooms I learned about the technologies that reporters use to identify news stories, the steps that they take to coordinate their reporting with others who work in their newsroom (editors, supervisors, camera operators, and other reporters), the ways that reporters process source texts into news articles, and how they think about aligning their writing activities with the overall vision of their news organization. While I started the project with the hope that I would be able to conduct extended institutional ethnographic observations in newsrooms and watch reporters' newswork over extended periods of time, it was challenging to connect with newsmakers who could accommodate this kind of ethnographic access. Due to reporters' hectic and often irregular work schedules, their concerns about confidentiality, and desire to speak freely about their newswork, reporters often requested that we meet outside of their workplace and invited me to join them at their local coffee shop for our interviews. This IE of news production is based on reporters' detailed descriptions of their work in interviews and fieldnotes from occasions when I was able to hold interviews in newsrooms.

The field of newsroom ethnography can broadly be understood to have developed in two waves. Sociologists who conducted the first wave of newsroom studies in the 1950s were mostly concerned with identifying the routines and orders of newsrooms to produce generalizable descriptions of how news is made (Usher 2014, 21). Early ethnographies of news production concentrated on editorial "gate-keepers" (White 1950) and the social structure of newsrooms (Breed 1955). In the 1970s studies focused largely on the ways that reporters rely on "official" authoritative sources who reliably provide information to reporters on a regular and timely basis. It has been widely noted that while journalists' connections to official sources enable them to satisfy the professional demand for quick, "impartial," and "objective news content" (Gans 1979), they also "produce a systematically structured over-accessing to the media of those in powerful and privileged institutional positions" (Hall et al. 1978, 58). These studies were significant because they illuminated how news tends to reproduce status quo definitions of social reality that reporters' "accredited sources" provide.

Since the mid-2000s, sociologists have studied how journalists' routines and work processes have changed in the digital age (Usher 2014, 21). Ethnographers have called attention to how journalists adjust to the demands that accompany digital news platforms, such as a 24/7 newscycle and an environment that demands more interactive engagement with readers (5). Studies have also highlighted the challenges, constraints, and pressures that journalists face as they incorporate novel technologies into their organizational workflow of news production (Anderson 2013; Batsell 2015; Brock 2013; Broersma and Peters 2012; Klinenberg 2005; Mitchelstein and Boczkowski 2009; Phillips 2014; Quandt 2008; Ryfe 2012; Steense and Ahva 2015).

The burgeoning crisis facing contemporary journalism is well established, and recent ethnographic studies of newsrooms have helped illustrate the economic, technological, and cultural challenges that news organizations are confronting (Almiron 2010; Barnett 2009; Fuller 2010; Levy and Nielsen 2010; Reinardy 2011). For example, journalism scholars have called attention to ways that print news production in the digital age is defined by radical uncertainty and marked by audience fragmentation, falling print circulation, the decline of the advertising model, dismal online advertising profits, and shrinking subscription revenues (Bell 2016; Saridou, Lia-Paschalia, and Veglis 2017; Usher 2018; Zelizer 2017). Studies show that in response to their precarious economic circumstances, news organizations have had to become more profit conscious and have been forced to reinvent themselves.

For many news organizations, reinvention takes the form of implementing "convergence models" to restructure their business strategies (Mitchelstein and Boczkowski 2009; Zhang 2012). The concept of convergence in journalism has many interpretations and definitions (Kolodzy 2006, 4); however, it generally refers to "the coming together of once-separate media in a digital, networked environment – in online journalism" (Pavlik 2001, 38). The Infotendcias Group (2012, 29–30) adds to an understanding of media convergence as a complex process that affects the production of news in myriad ways:

> Convergence journalism is a multidimensional process which, facilitated by the widespread implementation of digital communication technologies, affects the technological, business, professional, and editorial aspects of the media, fostering the integration of tools, spaces, working methods, and languages that were previously separate, in such a way that journalists can write contents to be distributed via multiple platforms.

This definition illuminates how convergence models operate at various levels of news organizations. At its core, convergence can be understood as a management strategy that news organizations adopt in order to keep labour costs down and to increase the output and efficiency of the news production process. The shift towards convergence means that news organizations reduce resource spending as they employ fewer reporters who are expected to cover more news topics across a range of news platforms. Thus, convergence models come to bear in significant ways on a news organization's business scheme, professional approach, resources, and news content (Doyle 2013; Klinenberg 2005; Lawson-Borders 2003; Quinn 2004; Saridou, Lia-Paschalia, and Veglis 2017).

Convergence journalism is a global phenomenon. Studies have documented how news organizations around the world have reinvented themselves as multimedia companies and highlighted how such a shift comes to bear on journalists' work. Like the journalists I spoke with in Canada for this project, ethnographic studies of convergence journalism in other jurisdictions emphasize the challenges that reporters face as they implement integrated newsrooms, simultaneously produce content for several channels (such as print, news websites, and social media), and engage in cross-distribution (Menke et al. 2019, 946). Scholars understand convergence journalism to be part of a broader, international "convergence culture" (Jenkins 2006; Menke et al. 2019, 946). As Menke and colleagues explain, convergence journalism "is not only defined by the ongoing global technological convergence of media platforms and technologies, but also 'represents a society-wide cultural shift affecting audiences, media, and corporations'" (Jenkins 2006, 3; Menke et al. 2019, 946).

In the Canadian context, a great deal of journalism now occurs under conditions of convergence. In 2017, the Standing Committee on Canadian Heritage released a report on the impact of technology on local and regional news. The report shows that the Canadian media industry is the most highly concentrated of any major comparable country in the world. In 2016, data showed that just three main groups (Postmedia, Transcontinental, Torstar) owned close to 66 per cent of all daily newspapers (Fry 2017, 53). Fewer sources of information means less original reporting, less investigative journalism, and less contact with local communities (55). The convergence of Canadian media corporations has resulted in significant staff layoffs; more than 16,500 jobs were lost in the media sector between 2008 and 2017 (56). Like many sectors, these precarious conditions were exacerbated by the COVID-19 pandemic. In 2020 alone, 67 Canadian media outlets closed temporarily or permanently and over 1,200 jobs were lost permanently, along with many more temporary layoffs (Wechsler 2021). Such staffing cuts have been said to negatively impact journalists' ability "to cover or investigate stories and to deliver the reporting that Canadians rely on to fully participate in a democracy" (Fry 2017, 56).

Newsroom ethnographies and studies of convergence journalism are useful for illustrating how the shifting structural conditions of contemporary journalism significantly shape journalists' everyday work. A unique contribution of this institutional ethnographic study of newswork in the digital era, is that it shows how writing for digital news shapes public knowledge of the issue of HIV criminalization in particular. In so doing, it prompts critical questions about the broader social implications of digital news production processes.

Digital News Metrics

A close look at reporters' newswork under the conditions of digital convergence journalism reveals that their everyday work is closely tied to the work that people do in other sites. In one sense, anticipating and aligning with the everyday practices of people across disparate locations has always been a defining characteristic of news production work. For instance, one way to understand newswork is as an exercise in aligning with and connecting to the news consumption practices and expectations of news audiences (Ananny and Finn 2020, 1600). For centuries news organizations have sought to efficiently coordinate news production routines with news consumption practices through a deeply engrained beat structure. Beat reporting refers to news organizations structuring the social environment they cover by organizing specialized (beat) reporters to cover specific subjects or geographic areas (Magin and Maurer 2019). Since the end of the nineteenth century this deepseated beat structure has meant that "news happened where journalists were pre-positioned, publishers and advertisers had economic interests, and audiences expected news to be" (160).

As reporters' accounts of their newswork in the next chapter illustrate, economic constraints that news organizations are encountering mean that the beat structure is not as stable as it once was. However, a recent "infrastructural turn" in media studies highlights ways that the organizational structure of anticipatory journalism has endured and expanded across a wide range of sites (Ananny and Finn 2020, 1601; Braun 2015; Parks and Starosielski 2015; Plantin and Punathambekar 2019). Today, digital news reporters not only align their newswork with the routines and practices of their newsroom, but also with "largely invisible digital infrastructures," including software data and technologies, social media, platform design, data, algorithms, and artificial intelligence (J. van Dijk, Poell, and de Wall 2018). These forces have a tremendous influence on how online news is predicted, defined, produced, circulated, interpreted, and acted upon.

My interviews with digital reporters helped me to understand how these kinds of technologies have materially changed how journalists can work. This was especially clear when reporters described how digital analytic dashboards (produced by corporations like Google, Adobe, Chartbeat, and others) that display real-time data about how online audiences are consuming news content hook their work into a highly competitive digital market. These technologies constantly confront reporters with quantified representations of how audiences are consuming the news they write as they track what content audiences like, share, comment on, and spend time with (Ananny and Finn 2020, 1609). Reporters I spoke with have an acute understanding of how this data is enmeshed in the market relations of digital news. As Ananny and Finn describe, "while online news organizations earn revenue through a mix of subscriptions, memberships, grants, and crowdfunding, the economics of news require them to aggressively pursue, monitor, retain, and predict audiences' attention on their websites and on social media platforms and apps … so that they might identify potential markets for personalized coverage and targeted advertisements" (2020, 1609).

As these digital analytic infrastructures coordinate the market economy of online news, they also come to bear on reporters' everyday newswork, and in turn, shape news content. Studies show that reporters' work with this data informs how they select news topics, write headlines and leads for news stories, and structure their publication rhythms. As noted in the next chapter, the reporters I spoke with explain that the emphasis that news organizations place on audience data also leads them to grapple with foundational components of newswork, such as assessments of newsworthiness and the professional ethics of journalism itself (Ananny and Finn 2020, 1609; Christin 2020; Petre 2015). Recognizing the powerful ways that digital news metrics gear into newswork is important for gaining a broader, more relational perspective on the social organization of newswork. Reporters' accounts of their everyday work in the coming chapters invite us to understand the newsroom as a site where practices and values that originate outside of the realm of journalism ultimately align with and routinize newswork (Ananny and Finn 2020, 1610).

In the next chapter I look more closely at the social organization of digital newswork by introducing readers to reporters who produce digital news content. As reporters describe how they arrange their work schedules to keep up with the never-ending demand for eye-catching news stories, we can begin to recognize how the ruling relations of digital news production set reporters up to produce sensational news content about HIV criminalization.

Chapter Two

The Everyday Work of Writing for Digital News

To learn about how news stories about HIV criminalization are produced, I spoke with news reporters like Shawn. Shawn meets me on the street below the skyscraper in which he works as a beat reporter for *The Daily Journal*. He's chatty while he finishes his smoke break but grows quiet as he leads me into the lobby, up the elevator to the newsroom floor, and into the cafeteria. The whole city is visible from up here. Maybe the view is especially striking on this sunny November afternoon, or perhaps I just appreciate it more because lately, as I try to wrap up fieldwork for my dissertation, I've been shut indoors pouring over freshly typed interview transcripts. I was initially hesitant to speak with Shawn for the thought of having to add the subsequent interview transcript to the stack of data that needs to be combed through. However, my friend Neil convinced me that meeting with Shawn would be well worth my time. Neil met Shawn years ago when the two were undergraduates working for their student newspaper. Shawn was the paper's editor. According to Neil, even as an undergraduate student, Shawn was unmistakeably serious about writing the news and seemed to fit the mould of the old-school beat reporter: his relentless pacing of their office hallways in the hours before a deadline, his curt phone calls with sources, and his relentless hunts for new story leads reminded Neil of the reporters typically depicted in newsroom dramas on screen.

Now Shawn sits across from me, and I can't help but agree that he looks as though he arrived at our interview from central casting, complete with the wardrobe of crumpled denim shirt that he wore with the sleeves rolled up, ballcap perched high on his head, and bleary eyes that he explained had to do with a string of recent late nights at his computer. His low, guarded voice, and the way he leaned in closer to me from across the table when answering questions, gave the impression that he had experience discussing sensitive matters with clandestine sources. His posture made our interview feel important.

When I met Shawn in 2017, he and his colleagues were facing the daily grind of producing news at a time when the public's trust in mainstream news was dwindling. The concept of "fake news" was rampant in public discourse at the time, thanks to a newly elected president's attack on professional news media. Just three weeks before I met Shawn, Collins Dictionary named "fake news" as their word of the year for 2017 – defined as "false, often sensational, information disseminated under the guise of news reporting" (Hunt 2017). It is, however, important to note that public trust in the mainstream press was dwindling prior to the US election in 2017, and the decline has persisted in subsequent years (Petre 2021, 4). For example, a recent study found that 49 per cent of Canadians believe journalists "are purposely trying to mislead people by saying thing things they know are false or gross exaggerations" (Fenlon 2021).

Communication scholars tend not to locate the cause of misinformation in the press in the activities or perspectives of individual journalists, and instead suggest that the rapid circulation of misinformation in mainstream news has to do with "the current media ecosystem" and how "the media's dependence on social media, analytics and metrics, sensationalism, novelty over newsworthiness, and clickbait makes them vulnerable to such media manipulation" (Marwick and Lewis 2017). This chapter is about how that news media ecosystem is put together, and more specifically, ways that environment organizes and perpetuates the production of sensational news stories about HIV criminalization.

Before homing in on the issue of HIV criminalization, it is worth recounting one of Shawn's first experiences reporting sensational news. He tells a story about how the pressure that reporters face to produce a "quick hit" piece of news content can cause one to "get burned":

> We need to get burned ... I got burned once and I don't do that [write quick news stories] anymore ... There was a report of a video of a shark, it was right at the start of my career, there was this YouTube video of a shark in Lake Ontario ... I got sent the video and my editor asked, "can you write something quick on this?" So, I called the restaurant on the island and they told me, "I'm not sending my kids in the lake and we're all really freaked out about this." I called some other people and they said they had seen the video and were all freaked out about this. There's these two fishermen on the dock and then this shark comes out and takes their catch and they all freak out. I couldn't find the people, I couldn't reach, this is

what haunts me, is that I couldn't speak to the people who made the video or the fisherman in the video, nobody seemed to know them. I write this story, nothing about a shark, like I kind of glossed over, it could be a shark, nobody knows what it is but this video has really freaked out these people on this little island and that's the story. It's really big and we quoted a marine biologist who says, "I don't think that's a shark, I don't know what that it is, but it's possible, they have come up the St. Lawrence before." Anyway, it turns out it was a Bell Media gag, like it was part of a promo for their "Shark Week" on Discovery Channel. And I was fucking livid. I had just started my job here, I was so mad. We never really said there was a shark, anyway, it just is like, that situation, that like quick hit, like, it's, you're so prone to error when you're under that kind of pressure, that I'd rather just screw it and say fuck it because it's [reporting misinformation is] so possible.

Shawn's story encapsulates a lot of what I came to recognize as the hallmarks of reporters' daily newswork. For one, his account starts to show how the short timeline to produce a "quick hit" type of news story organizes reporters' work routines. In the passage above, Shawn acknowledges that the pressure to produce the "quick hit" made him "prone to error." His description of his newswork practice also directs attention to how sources that reporters rely on shape news content. This interview segment is a reminder of just how porous the line between news producers and news audiences is in the age of the smartphone. The main source of Shawn's news story is not an event he witnessed firsthand, but an online video that was spreading fast across social media. As I will describe throughout this chapter, the work that reporters do to produce online news is often characterized by activities to process digital source texts into news content as quickly as possible. There are important ways that the social organization of writing for digital news positions reporters to produce sensational news stories.

My institutional ethnography of online news is based on interviews I carried out with twenty-one journalists in which I asked them about the routine steps they take to produce a news report. Throughout this book I refer to reporters' everyday work activities as "newswork." Journalism scholarship has established a register of activities that characterize what is commonly recognized as "newswork" (Gans 1979; Tuchman 1978; Zelizer 2017, 31). This set of practices is ever shifting. For example, typesetting skills of the print room have given way to contemporary demands for journalists to possess general and broad digital media production skills. As we see in this chapter, within the digital newsroom journalists' newswork routines include conducting online research to locate stories, pitching stories to news editors, identifying sources to interview, finding digital source texts (newswires, press releases, social media content, and other news articles), transferring segments of source texts into news articles, and producing digital news texts that can be quickly and efficiently spread across multiple formats.

Each of the twenty-one interviews that I conducted helped me to better understand the social world of contemporary newswork. The reporters I spoke with do their work from within varied work settings and for diverse news agencies. I spoke to staff reporters who work in the newsrooms of major Canadian newspapers and smaller regional newspapers; freelance journalists who write for free, alternative publications; and others who work for newswires that produce news content that is disseminated in newspapers across the country. Interviews with this range of journalists helped to reveal how particular social relations of news production shape reporters' newswork.

This empirical account of how reporters' newswork is socially organized surfaces the extent to which their everyday work practices consist of activating texts[1] and traces how the highly textual character of reporters' newswork is coordinated by relations of commercialization and generalist reporting associated with convergence journalism. As the experiences of reporters who are featured in this chapter demonstrate, a work environment in which reporters are required to rapidly and continuously produce news stories that will be widely consumed by online readers is likely to produce sensational accounts of topics such as HIV criminalization.

This chapter unfolds in three parts. In the first section, I display a typical news story about HIV criminalization. The news article exhibits the characteristics of the crime story genre that has consistently structured news reports of HIV criminalization for decades. In addition, the news report shows how mainstream news media regularly link race, migration status, crime, and HIV serostatus so as to circulate representations of racialized people living with HIV, especially those who are

---

1 I use the phrase "activate" texts to refer to ways that people's work with texts in their local work processes enters their activities into courses of action and work being done in other sites and at other times (D.E. Smith 2005, 170). Institutional ethnographers employ the language of "activating" texts in order to explore how texts operate as coordinators of ruling relations. As Dorothy Smith describes, "recognizing texts as people activate them in their work, as they occur, makes possible the expansion of ethnography beyond the local to explore and explicate institutional order. It makes visible the presence of institutional relations in the everyday of people's lives" (D.E. Smith 2005, 169).

newcomers to Canada, as dangerous "Others." I present and discuss the news article not as a prelude to an analysis of representation but as a jumping off point for an analysis of the social world of news production. In the second section of the chapter, I ground my analysis of the news in reporters' descriptions of their everyday work activities. Most notably, I show that journalists' newswork consists primarily of text-processing activities that characterize "writing for digital news." I conclude the chapter by reflecting on the potential scope of IE for making sense of the social organization of newswork.

The Surface of News Reports of HIV Criminalization

Before I turn to look closely at journalists' everyday newswork practices, it is useful for readers to have a clear sense of some of the defining features of news reports about HIV criminalization. When considering the corpus of news coverage on this topic as a whole, it is essential to emphasize that HIV activists have voiced deep concerns about how HIV criminalization is portrayed in the press for decades. Since the first charges related to alleged HIV non-disclosures were laid in 1989, activists have called attention to common deeply stigmatizing and objectifying tropes that shape news stories about HIV and the criminal law. I learned about the corpus of Canadian newspaper articles about HIV criminalization through collaborative work on a community report that colleagues and I published in late 2016 entitled *"Callous, Cold and Deliberately Duplicitous": Racialization, Immigration and the Representation of HIV Criminalization in Canadian Mainstream Newspapers*. The goal of the report was to provide empirical evidence for activists' claims that African, Caribbean, and Black (ACB) people living with HIV are overrepresented and negatively portrayed in Canadian newspaper stories about HIV non-disclosure cases.

The report examined each of the 1,680 English-language Canadian newspaper articles published about HIV non-disclosure criminal cases in Canada written between 1989 and 2015. Our quantitative study confirmed that people from ACB communities who face criminal charges related to HIV non-disclosure are in fact drastically overrepresented in news coverage. While men from these communities account for only 15 per cent of defendants charged, they are the focus of 61 per cent of newspaper coverage (Mykhalovskiy et al. 2016). In addition to conducting a quantitative analysis that spoke to the issue of the overrepresentation of ACB communities in news stories, we also produced a discursive analysis that highlighted forms of language that circulated in articles to objectify people living with HIV (especially African, Caribbean, and

Black men living with HIV) as dangerous and blameworthy people who pose a threat to public health and, more broadly, the imagined Canadian nation.

As part of our discursive analysis, we produced a detailed description of a news report published in the *Globe and Mail* by Canadian journalist Christie Blatchford on 22 October 2008 headlined, "HIV-Positive Man Was 'Actively Involved' Patient Concerned with His Well-Being, Specialist Testifies." The 1,042-word article reports on the criminal trial of a person facing charges related to HIV non-disclosure who I will refer to as J.A. (Blatchford 2008). We selected this particular article because it encapsulates many of the common tropes that contribute to the corpus of news discourse about HIV criminalization materializing as a collection of objectifying, sensational, and stigmatizing crime stories. Here, I draw on this description from our community report to underline some of the most prominent discursive trends that we recognized in news coverage of HIV criminalization.

For instance, the most noticeable feature of the article is that it is written as a crime story. One of the characteristics of news coverage that became obvious as we reviewed news stories about HIV criminalization in 2016 is that the mainstream press has consistently reported on HIV non-disclosure as a type of crime story since the first charges were laid in Canada in the late 1980s (Mykhalovskiy et al. 2016). Media scholars interested in representation often understand crime stories as a type of media frame (Entman 2003; Gitlan 1980). Studies of news media frames attend to how news coverage "select[s] some aspects of a perceived reality and make[s] them more salient in a communicating text" (Entman 1993, 52; Jiwani and Young 2006; Ryan, Carragee, and Meinhofer 2001, 176). For example, studies of the crime story frame show that it regularly emphasizes sensational, violent aspects of crimes (Altheide 2003). Important critical race studies have also pointed to ways that news reports that are framed as crime stories contribute to the criminalization of racialized people by consistently depicting racialized people as particularly violent and threatening (Entman 1992, 1994; Jiwani 2006; Oliver 2003).

In this book, I employ the concept of the "crime story genre" as opposed to the crime story frame. While studies of media frames attend to the content of news discourse, the concept of "genre" is used in analyses that understand discourse as a type of social activity (van Dijk 2018, 232). Teun van Dijk (2018) describes that "genres are defined in terms of the properties of the communicative situation or *context*, such as Who, When, Where, for whom, and How the discourse is used, as well as by their style of meanings" (229; emphasis in the original).

He goes on to explain that genres are communicative situations that may be characterized by categories such as time period, institution, participants, and social roles.

A defining feature of the stable and consistent crime story genre about HIV criminalization is that news reports are structured by the institutional logic, relevancies, and routine events of the criminal legal system (Mykhalovskiy et al. 2021b). In our review of Canadian newspaper articles about HIV non-disclosure criminal cases, we referred to this characteristic of crime genre reporting about HIV non-disclosure as "criminal justice time." The notion of criminal justice time emphasizes how news coverage is coordinated by the routine events that sequence the criminal legal processing of a case: news written in this way reports on a standardized sequence of events through which HIV non-disclosure criminal cases proceed (stories are published *when* a person is arrested, *when* a bail hearing is held, *when* people testify in court, etc.) (793). While other types of news articles, such as editorials and opinion pieces, are published about HIV criminalization, the vast majority of news articles in the corpus that we reviewed addressed a specific case of HIV non-disclosure that was before the courts.

This sequencing of stories is apparent in Blatchford's reporting on HIV criminalization. Between October 2008 and April 2009, Blatchford wrote nine stories about J.A., each of which reports on a development in the criminal-legal processing of the case against him. This patterning of crime genre stories is significant because it works to objectify J.A. as a criminal subject, functions to provide a discourse that reinforces an understanding of HIV non-disclosure as a criminal offence, and creates a stock of reporting that invites news readers to think about HIV non-disclosure in this way. When news stories are coordinated by the standard processing of a criminal-legal case, readers only come to know about HIV non-disclosure as a crime and only hear about the person accused of not disclosing their HIV-positive status in relation to the crime they are being charged with.

Another common feature of criminal justice time reporting on HIV criminalization that we recognized in Blatchford's article has to do with how news reports regularly portray African, Caribbean, and Black men in negative and stereotypical ways. A common way that this occurs is through news reports that link representations of racialized difference and migration status with constructions of moral blameworthiness (Mykhalovskiy et al. 2021b, 789–90). It is worth noting, for instance, that Blatchford substitutes the descriptor "the Ugandan immigrant" in place of J.A.'s name as she introduces the criminal charges that are being laid against him in order to produce J.A. as a dangerous, threatening

"Other." This otherness is also regularly constructed through the use of photographs and frequent reference to him as "Ugandan-born" and as a "refugee" (Mykhalovskiy et al. 2016, 44).

Finally, Blatchford's article about J.A. provides an example of how news coverage of HIV criminalization often uses expert testimony given at criminal trials to frame people living with HIV as morally blameworthy and reckless people (Mykhalovskiy et al. 2016, 44). News stories rarely feature the voices, experiences, perspectives, or expertise of people living with HIV or organizations that represent them and instead rely on what other experts say about people facing criminal charges, most often in ways that objectify people living with HIV by underlining their moral blameworthiness. It is common for reporters to piece together parts of testimonies from public health authorities, physicians, and medical experts that Crown prosecutors introduce to try to establish that a defendant is guilty of a crime, with their own narrative accounts of what was said at trial. In Blatchford's article, for example, the headline and the bulk of the article rely on testimony from an infectious disease specialist at the criminal trial as a way to produce a narrative about a morally abject person (45). For instance, the article consists of direct quotes from the specialist named in the article to highlight the number of times J.A. visited the specialist's clinic, J.A.'s reluctance to begin taking antiretroviral medication, and to describe how J.A. "was actively involved and very concerned about his health" (Blatchford 2008). The article uses this testimony to establish a story about an irresponsible person living with HIV.

The tenor of news articles about HIV criminalization has shifted in recent years, thanks in large part to the highly committed and strategic media work of HIV activists. Chapter 5 details ways that advocates have worked to ensure that their critiques of HIV criminalization are included in news coverage of the topic and mobilize discourses that counter the stigmatizing and sensational pattern of reporting exemplified in Blatchford's piece. Unfortunately, problematic, sensational patterns persist in some news coverage of HIV criminalization. This was the case, for instance, in coverage of the criminal trial of a thirty-one-year-old man in Edmonton who was charged with aggravated sexual assault related to HIV non-disclosure in 2021.

Articles, such as one entitled "Crown Drops Charges against Edmonton Man Accused of Passing HIV to Sex Partner; Defense Says Handling of Health Issue in Justice System 'Deplorable,'" display an enduring and troubling standardization of news coverage of this issue. For one, the article includes a mugshot-style photo of the person (described in court testimony included in the article as "a Black trans sex worker") facing criminal charges and relies heavily on information from a police press release. This is particularly confounding, considering that the article also includes quotations from HIV advocates and the defence lawyer criticizing police for publishing this personal information about the person facing charges in the first place.

There are also concerning inaccuracies in the news headline and the article itself. For example, aggravated sexual assault charges in this context have to do with the non-disclosure of one's HIV-positive status, not "passing HIV to a sex partner." The article also describes that the man is "accused of passing the AIDS virus," despite the fact AIDS is not a transmittable disease. HIV can progress to AIDS; however, current treatment is highly effective in preventing transmission, suppressing HIV, and preventing progression to AIDS (HIV Legal Network 2020). The article's reference to the "infecting" of a fifty-nine-year-old man with HIV is also outdated and stigmatizing terminology. The language of a "person or people living with HIV" is now much more common and widely preferred. The types of inaccuracies and stigmatizing language that have structured news coverage of this topic for decades and echo throughout this piece from 2021 are cause for alarm. At a time when activists are making monumental strides towards law reform, articles such as this one instruct readers to cling to some of the most outdated and harmful discursive connections between HIV, race, gender, crime, and risk – or at least obscure the many reasons that there is an urgent need for legal reform on HIV criminalization.

There are many ways sociologists concerned with HIV stigma, processes of criminalization, and the way that media act as an important source of public information about health and law might develop a critical analysis of the enduring trends in these articles. For instance, one could situate these news texts within a broader study of representation that adds to understandings of how meaning is given and how power and knowledge intersect in dominant explanations of crime (Brock, Glasbeek, and Murdocca 2014; Henry and Tator 2002). A critical researcher might pursue a study of news content that adds to the work of Canadian scholars who have drawn on the work of Stuart Hall to show how race and racism are deeply embedded in media representations of crime, and emphasize how racialized people are consistently represented as "others" who exist outside of and as threats to the imagined community of Canada (Chan and Chunn 2014; Jiwani and Young 2006; Lawson 2014). One might also draw on the articles to extend the research literature on media representations of HIV criminalization in particular. As I have started to show, these news reports exemplify many of the common themes identified in empirical reviews of news coverage of the issue. For instance, Blatchford's piece typifies how press coverage consistently relies on a sharp criminal–victim dichotomy, constructs Black men as hypersexual and predatory, inflates HIV risks, represents Black men as "foreign" others, and silences the perspectives of defendants (Lupton 1999; McKay et al. 2011; Mykhalovskiy et al. 2021b; Persson and Newman 2008).

My study of news coverage of HIV criminalization in Canada is informed by this rich collection of literature. I am particularly indebted to critical race scholars who help me to understand these news texts as artefacts of a standard genre of crime reporting that establishes connections between race and crime and mediates the public's understanding of "criminals." I work to extend this trajectory of media research in this book, but I take a slightly different approach. Rather than attending to the content of news texts, this institutional ethnographic study shifts analysis towards the work that reporters do to produce a news story and the social contexts in which reporters write.

The Everyday Work of Journalists

At the outset of my fieldwork, I expected that my research would take me to the gritty everyday and every night worlds of journalists that circulate in popular depictions of news production. I wanted a front-row seat to witness how the tension builds as intrepid reporters clack away on their keyboards to file a breaking story just ahead of their deadline. I anticipated that I'd be privy to dramatic moments in which reporters go head-to-head with editors to convince them that the investigative piece they've been toiling over for months *is* ready for print. That powerful scene from the film *Spotlight* in which a leather jacket–clad Mark Ruffalo implores Michael Keaton to run their story that exposes the massive scandal and cover-up within the local Catholic Archdiocese comes to mind: "It's time, Robby! It's time!"

Over the years that I researched and wrote this book there were numerous examples of influential, longform, investigative Canadian journalism that spoke truth to power: David Bruser and Jayme Poisson reported on the Ontario Government's cover-up of buried mercury upstream of Grassy Narrows First Nation; Sara Mojtehedzadeh went undercover in an industrial bakery where a young worker had recently died to reveal the abhorrent conditions that temporary workers face; the investigative CBC series *Deadly Force* built a national database of Canadians killed in police-involved fatalities; and Tom Cardoso's two-year inquiry into the Canadian prison system uncovered systemic bias against Black and Indigenous inmates.

These journalistic endeavours are just a few examples to illustrate that when media organizations devote time and resources to support the work of talented reporters, the press can uphold its position as an integral check on those in positions of power and expose systemic violence. At the same time, the newsrooms that I visited and the reporters I spoke with also brought a much different picture of journalism into view. There are two main ways that the everyday work of reporters that I observed working in the context of convergence journalism diverged from what I expected to find in newsrooms. First, writing for digital news is a much more collaborative type of writing practice than I anticipated. Though most newspaper articles are headed by a byline that attributes the text's authorship to one or two journalists, this study shows that journalists' work practices are part of an extended dynamic dialogue premised largely on processing talk and text from various digital sources into multiple digital formats. Second, popular representations of journalists often focus on their beat work – the way that they "pound the pavement" to access sources and leads for news stories. However, reporters I spoke with regularly described their work to select, source, and research stories as a desk-top, text-based activity. These two features of journalism that resonated throughout my interviews with reporters helped me to understand the work of writing for digital news.

Close attention to the work practices of journalists is central to this book. The concept of "work" is commonly used in institutional ethnographic research as a term that locates inquiry in the "actualities of what people do on a day-to-day basis" (Mykhalovskiy and McCoy 2002, 24; D.E. Smith 1987, 166). According to Dorothy Smith, this means beginning research in people's descriptions of their work – "what people do that requires some effort, that they mean to do, and that involves some acquired competence" (165). Building on contributions from institutional ethnographers who have extended the general concept of "work" to explore the social organization of particular empirical sites (for example, see Mykhalovskiy and McCoy 2002 on "health work") I use the concept of "newswork" to direct attention towards the wide range of activities that journalists do to produce a news report.

This section of the chapter that examines the everyday work of journalists proceeds in two parts. First, in an effort to make the everyday work activities of journalists visible, I draw on two interviewees' accounts of their typical workday. One interviewee, Alex, is a young daily news reporter at News Centre. His descriptions of his work illustrate how journalists access, process, and repurpose an array of talk and text in order to produce news content that can be spread across multiple platforms at once. The other journalist, Sarah, worked for Urban News as the agency's web editor. Her account offers insights into how online news happens and shows how news editors process, arrange, and filter digital texts so as to ensure a constant flow of "fresh" news content. Together, these accounts demonstrate that journalists' newswork can be understood primarily as a practice of text production. In the second part of this section, I move to locate journalists' work practices in the actual relations by which they are organized. In particular, I put forward an empirical description of how the social world of news production is organized by the relations of convergence journalism.

Feeding, Sending, Isolating, and Chopping Daily News

As was the case with many of the reporters I interviewed, it took several rounds of emails and text messages with Alex to arrange a time to meet that fit the hectic schedule that he navigates as a daily news reporter. After a couple of weeks of correspondence, Alex suggested we meet early on a Wednesday morning at a downtown Toronto Starbucks. As I rode the Dundas streetcar east, on a bright but brutally cold morning, my phone buzzed with a series of text messages that helped me get a sense of Alex's energy and enthusiasm before I met him in person. It became clear that his proficiency for relaying news updates extended outside the newsroom and into his personal interactions as well. His messages asked if we could meet in the west-end instead (his plans had changed and it would be easier for him to ride his bike there), questioned if our new meeting spot had Wi-Fi and if he should bring his laptop, and offered updates such as "ooooh you're early! Just brushing my teeth, then coming over!" It was clear from the outset of our interview that Alex loves his job a great deal and that he finds his work as a reporter to be consistently exciting, stimulating, and challenging. At points during our conversation he became so enthusiastic while describing his work that he had to stop himself, take a breath, and begin again. Since our interview, I have heard Alex file news reports on the radio a number of times, and I have been struck by how much his commanding, deep, and deliberate news radio voice differs from the eager, brisk, and bouncy way that he spoke when we met.

In addition to being difficult to pin down for an interview, another characteristic that Alex shared with many reporters I spoke with is that he was much younger than I expected he would be. Throughout my fieldwork I learned that daily news in Canada is largely produced by young reporters, often fresh from journalism school. Industry insiders suggest that in an age of resource scarcity, younger reporters typically demand less pay and are more willing to work longer hours (Bilton 2015). At the same time, young journalists are regularly expected to be "change agents" who foster innovation and stretch existing boundaries in the profession (Broersma and Singer 2020).

I first came to know about Alex's work while I was interviewing Gabe, one of Alex's colleagues at News Centre. Gabe mentioned Alex while he was trying to articulate the intense pressures that young reporters confront in contemporary newsrooms. He described that Alex "has to produce for TV, radio, web, sometimes four files in a matter of two days, that's a lot." Gabe saw Alex as the sort of young reporter that editors will

sic to the wolves every day ... because they're young and inexperienced, you know, they're eager and so we say, "go get it," and they have to file [news stories] on two or three platforms and there's only so much time ... they don't have a lot of time to ... really understand something and you know, you're only jumping in on the story for a day or two because the resources aren't there.

My interview with Alex offered important insight into how he organizes his everyday work activities in order to balance the multiple tasks that Gabe described. At the very outset of our interview Alex explained that his everyday work requires multiple skill sets and forms of knowledge:

I work as a reporter at News Centre in French. I primarily work in TV, but I also do radio and web. I work, my beat is business but I've also done stories about public health and so I've touched on HIV, PrEP, that sort of thing. I also do stories about education and francophone affairs. Primarily my work is in French, but I also do pitch stories on the English side for Toronto or national.

This description was important for my initial understanding of the variety of practices that comprise Alex's newswork. For example, this segment shows that Alex's work activities traverse multiple languages, media platforms, story-telling techniques, and news topics. Another important aspect of this passage is Alex's reference to pitching stories, which offers insight into how he is positioned within the structure of the news agency. It is not as though Alex can independently select a topic and begin writing on his own accord. The process of writing a news story begins with Alex "pitching" ideas for a news story to an assignment producer. Alex explained that he arrives at the office each day with up to three pitches in mind, "then our assignment producer will be like, 'yes do this' … or 'no, that's a bad idea, here's another story' … but that's when our assignment producer will sort of give us a story, either something we've pitched or something else that's maybe in the news or there's been a press release." This segment starts to show that writing for digital news is an activity that is closely tied to the broader priorities and processes of a reporter's news agency. For instance, Alex's newswork requires him to write with an awareness of his editors' work practices, procedures, and sense of newsworthiness.

The pitch meetings that occur before Alex begins writing a news story are one way that he aligns his newswork with editorial processes. Alex also described how editors circulate data to regulate the content and form of his writing. Editors at News Centre regularly distribute data that quantifies how online readers engage with articles on the news agency's website. Alex described that he receives,

> usually weekly updates on "here are the top stories of the week, this has been the number of shares, clicks," there's different metrics … those are emailed out to everyone. So, everyone knows what stories worked, what didn't work. Interestingly sometimes the stories that were shared the most, had like ten second views, sometimes people see a headline and they'll share it without even reading the story. So that's another metric that we look at, like, okay well my story was maybe seventh on the list, but had a readership of about a minute, a minute thirty, so you know people actually spend more time in my story than the one that was shared the most. So obviously, you have to take into consideration all those different elements.

Alex explained that he understands the purpose of editors sharing this data is to encourage reporters to model their news stories on those that have been viewed and shared most widely online. Thus, his newswork not only involves having story ideas vetted by editors, it also centres on the effort to model his text production activities upon news texts that are understood by editors to be "the top stories of the week." Together, Alex's account of the pitch meeting and his description of how digital news metrics are circulated by editors, reinforce an understanding of writing for digital news as highly responsive to particular organizational priorities.

Alex's account of his typical workday also brought into view the extent to which his work to produce news content consists mainly of activating existing texts. He coordinates his daily work routine to ensure that he meets News Centre's demand for the production of a steady stream of news content that can be spread across multiple news platforms. To do so, Alex explained that he considers "every hour as a deadline" for producing and circulating news texts:

> It used to be like, oh you just have your six o'clock deadline or your four o'clock radio deadline but now we're just constantly producing 24-hour news, so I think of every hour as a deadline and I think about what can I provide every hour essentially ... Sometimes there are days when I'm like, the story is factual and accurate and everything, but I didn't add my personal ... how can I? I feel like I didn't make it as fun or interesting as it could have been in terms of the writing style and creativity and whatnot just because I didn't have time to go through everything and add little clips and edit. So sometimes I'm like, ugh, this story could have been so much better had I had time to go through everything.

Reporters I interviewed regularly historicized their experiences in newsrooms in a similar way to Alex. It was common for journalists to contrast the overwhelming speed at which news is produced in the digital era with what they understood to be the more deliberate routines of analogue newsrooms. In this passage, Alex describes the stress, apprehension, and frustration that he experiences as he works throughout the day to routinely produce a particular type of news text – a text that can be produced quickly, efficiently, and in step with the dizzying pace of digital news production. It is clearly challenging for Alex to square the organizational demand for the constant and rapid production of news texts with his vision of a sort of newswork that would allow him to insert his unique voice and writing style into a news text. We can see how the managerial expectation for consistent and efficient text production prevents Alex from expressing his personal journalistic voice.

As Alex described his everyday newswork, it became clear that his work centres not only on the constant and rapid production of texts, but on the production of a type of text that can be efficiently modified and repurposed by others in his news agency. Consider Alex's description of his typical workday:

> Okay, typical day ... I'll send out a bunch of emails, I'm looking for sources of people who are experts on the matter who can talk, I guess it depends on the story, but let's say I'm working on a public health story on vaccination. I'll try and line up interviews with government officials, experts on the matter, pharmacists or doctors or whatever, then I'll go out ... trying to squeeze in all those interviews, then I'm going out with my cameraman to all those different interviews. While I do all of this,

radio wants to be fed so I usually will send in a one-minute rant on my topic with a few interviews that I've done and we'll just sort of sum their ideas and produce a one-minute rant that's going to be played for a few radio newscasts in the afternoon. I usually send in the written form of my radio newscast to the web team, and then they'll sort of make a web version of that article. Yeah and then so I usually try to be back at the station [by] the latest at three o'clock because I want to give myself time to write, to go through my footage, my material, and then I write up a TV script, you know, based on the interview clips that I've isolated. Then I have to get that vetted by the senior producer for the TV show. Once it's vetted I go voice it in a radio booth ... So then I usually take my TV story, chop out a few parts ... If there's anything that's a developing element in that story, sometimes I'll save something for that story for the next morning and maybe something for web. Like write up a small, like, web article on part two of this story and leave it for the next morning. So that's an average day.

This segment helps bring into view the tremendous volume of texts that Alex produces during a typical workday. While we most often associate journalists' work with their complete, published, news article, Alex describes that writing for digital news is based on producing other texts, such as emails, interview questions, interview transcripts, short rants based on these interviews, written newscasts to be broadcast on the radio, written newscasts to be broadcast on television, and multiple iterations of web articles. One could draw on this interview segment to add to studies of news media production that examine how journalists identify expert sources, conduct interviews, or develop scripts for radio and television broadcasts. However, I include this passage here because it illuminates that writing for digital news is largely about processing, transferring, and repurposing texts.

For instance, in this passage, important steps in Alex's newswork routine (as described in the first part of this section) have already been completed. He has presumably already pitched the news story to an assignment producer, and he has likely reviewed what type of news stories have recently garnered the highest volume of web traffic online (another sort of text-processing activity). The next steps in his newswork, as featured in this account, bring two important features of his everyday text processing practices into view. First, this description starts to show that Alex's work is rooted in activities that process various texts and talk into his news article. For example, his first step is to access expert sources whose voices he can insert into his news text. This once again underlines that writing for digital news is not a univocal exercise, it is a sort of writing practice that one conducts in dialogue with the talk and text of authoritative sources.

The second significant aspect of Alex's account of his text production practice is that it shows how his work is geared into the routines of many other actors in his news agency, such as camera operators, radio producers, website editors, and television producers. His newswork is about processing texts into his news article, but it is also about producing texts that others in his news agency can process, repurpose, and use for various news formats. For example, notice that his day is mostly an exercise in *feeding* interview texts into radio broadcasts; *sending* the written form of the radio broadcast to a web team who will reshape it into an online article; *isolating* and *chopping* interview segments that can be *transferred* into the script of a television broadcast that a newscaster will read on the air; and, finally, all the while keeping abreast of developments in the news story in order to produce shorter web articles that keep an online news site replete with the most recent details. These work practices in which Alex processes and repurposes a common source text, such as an interview, and spreads it widely across various news platforms enable him to meet the organizational demand for a steady supply of news content.

While Alex's account helps to show how reporters process and reprocess various digital texts in order to produce digital news content, it is worth pausing to highlight the particularly significant role that interview work plays in the production of digital news. Mats Nylund (2011, 480) writes,

the reporter source interview is an extremely important part of news production, but has only rarely been the subject of academic research. Even in the late 1980s, Teun van Dijk (1988, 137) drew attention to the lack of this kind of research. According to him, "Much more empirical work is necessary about the discourse processing of source texts and their transformation into final news discourse." Years later, such research continues to be rare.

Here, Nyland (2011, 480) helps us to understand news interviews as a kind of "news-generating machine" – a particular type of social situation that elicits replies and statements from the interviewee that are turned into quotes and sound-bits, the crucial raw material of news stories. In cases when reporters I spoke with had time and space to conduct first-hand research as part of their newswork activities, interview work tended to structure their routines. For example, Justin is a freelance reporter who works for a community news organization. He described,

Literally the first thing I ever do when I approach a story, I've gotten my assignment from my editor, I open a new document, I write the name of the story, and then I list the basic voices that I want ... [for the story about a criminal HIV non-disclosure case] I sat down and I wrote that I had to attempt to contact the guy [facing criminal charges] himself or his lawyer, I had to get two institutional voices, an activist voice, the police, and public health. Before I knew who any of these people were, I had to write down that these were the voices I want in the story, and I went about filling those voices in.

This passage is interesting because it helps to show how source interviews structure Justin's entire news production process. His newswork is about locating and collecting sources who will reply to his questions and subsequently provide the raw material that he requires to produce a news text. What Justin's remarks suggest is that source interviews are different from the litany of other digital processing and reprocessing work that reporters do. From the time a story is assigned to a reporter to the point at which the news article is published, sources can inform reporters' knowledge of an issue and shape news content in significant ways. In chapter 4, I expand on how HIV advocates utilize news interviews as the basis for interventions into news content. For now, I want to present source interview work as an important type of text-processing work that reporters do.

Pulling News Stories

Alex's description of his newswork shows the extent to which writing for digital news consists of producing, processing, repurposing, and distributing texts. While his account displays how reporters isolate, chop, feed, and send texts to other platforms across their news agency, the locations at which these texts arrive remain out of view in Alex's description of his local, everyday world. In order to "enlarge the scope" of my understanding of news production, I wanted to talk with someone whose daily work activities centre on receiving and processing the sort of news content Alex produces (McCoy 2006, 704). Fortunately, Sarah, a friend of a friend, responded to an open call for interview participants that I posted on social media. Sarah and I met at a coffee shop close to her office after work one evening. A few months before we met, Sarah left her job as a web editor at Urban News and started working as a communication specialist at a non-profit organization. Before I turned my tape recorder on, Sarah described that she was very much enjoying the more stable work schedule and calmer pace of her new job.

When she was a web editor at Urban News, Sarah's workday consisted mainly of sifting through long streams of news stories on digital news wires and making decisions about which ones to post on the Urban News website. Her work also involved arranging the stories on the site's homepage. She headed the sort of web team that would receive Alex's article and, as he described, "make a web version of that article." Sarah's work activities exemplify the type of text-processing and repurposing practices that are central to writing for digital news. Sarah described her work in the following way:

> So, I was a web editor at Urban News. So that makes it seem like I had more decision-making power than I did, the title seems really lofty. But basically, a large portion of my day was just pulling news from the wire, so Canadian Press and a little bit of AP, mostly Canadian Press ... So, when I say like, pulling stories, it would come through the system and it was really just assigning it a headline because usually the headlines weren't really that great that would come automated, adding a photo, then deciding to put it on social media ... And then so when I did deal with original content it was editing that content for the web, proofreading, not really fact-checking because there was no time, but proofreading, putting it up, tweeting it out. That was really a large portion.

Looking closely at Sarah's account of her work practices brings into view a remarkable collection of text-processing and repurposing activities. Most notably, her editorial work was about "pulling" news stories from various news wires and processing them into news content for the agency's website. This processing work included steps to add or alter the story's headline, to add a photo to the story, and to review the text in order to correct for errors in form. Sarah's reference to there being "no time" to fact check, reinforces the rapid pace at which news is produced in contemporary newsrooms. These time constraints meant that for the most part, Sarah made minimal modifications to the texts that she processed into web content. As she described, her work consisted of "copy and pasting it pretty much. Maybe you would tweak it a bit ... but that's pretty much it, you weren't really changing content unless you noticed a spelling mistake they missed or something like that." Much like Alex, Sarah coordinated her newswork activities in order to produce news texts as quickly as possible and to fulfil her news agency's demand for a constant supply of news content.

Sarah's descriptions of her work also illuminate that her practice of "pulling news stories" was rooted in the exercise of quickly evaluating texts and assessing which ones ought to be included on the homepage. For example, she specifies in the segment above that some of the headlines she came across "weren't really that great." During our interview, it seemed challenging for Sarah to articulate how she evaluated texts, to explain precisely how she knew which stories to pull from the wire and process into web content, or to specifically define what characterized a newsworthy article. She described that many of the articles that came through the wire over the course of her eight-hour shift were clearly not relevant to her paper's readership. As she explained,

> it was kind of like picking, because a lot of the stuff we would have never have chosen to put up, so it would be like ... some random crime story from the States, and we'd be like, it doesn't really matter ... or like, a million sports stories that we don't need, something random like, I don't know, track and field, but it would all come through [the wire].

This segment begins to show how Sarah's newswork to pull stories and place them on the web was coordinated by her anticipation of how Urban News's online readership would receive the article. In this passage, it seems easy for her to pass over stories that have to do with events that occur outside the newspaper's geographic location or that report on events that would only interest a niche audience. Her newswork is about assessing news stories in terms of what content is relevant to a wide segment of readers and will, in turn, attract a high volume of online visitors to the website. Sarah stated that the criteria for what counted as newsworthy "was definitely very subjective to be able to pick what you thought was interesting or what you thought people would be interested in." As she described her work, she identified sources that she used as barometers to gauge what stories would interest a wide segment of readers and draw visitors to the homepage.

For example, Sarah's work regularly involved monitoring the webpages of other news agencies. Sarah explained that one of her colleagues "would see what [news story] was doing well elsewhere, it's like, oh do we have this story yet? Because it's actually doing really well over here. Maybe we should grab that." Sarah and her co-workers also watched social media feeds in a similar way: "I think if something for some reason exploded on Facebook I'd be like maybe we need to revisit where it's placed on our homepage." Checking social media was a central part of Sarah's work because often times social media would alert Sarah to an important news story before it came through on the news wires she was monitoring and looking to "pull" stories from. She described, "Sometimes you're waiting for something to come through [the wire]. Nowadays you see something that happens on Twitter and that happens before the wire comes through and so you're like, aahh when is this coming through [the wire]!?" Sarah's work to track news stories on competing organizations' homepages and on social media feeds displays a particular type of text-processing activity. Sarah repurposes online news stories as text devices that support her work to evaluate what news stories are relevant and likely to attract readers to the homepage that she coordinates as a web editor.

A primary way that Sarah worked to draw readers to the Urban News website was by constantly updating and maintaining a steady stream of "fresh" stories on the homepage. Over the course of her eight-hour shift Sarah made regular revisions to the stories that were featured on the homepage and the way that they were arranged: "depending on the day, I would say [the homepage would be refreshed] like twenty times, sometimes more … I would say, just like every half hour maybe." Sarah understood that a consistent flow of novel content on the homepage made it more likely that readers would visit the site multiple times throughout the day and, as she emphasized, "you want them to check back in." While Sarah was mostly responsible for the layout of the homepage, her supervisors would sometimes bypass her editorial work by scheduling news stories to "go live." Essentially, stories would be scheduled to "go live" in order to coordinate the layout of the Urban News homepage with the layout of the print version of the daily Urban News. As Sarah described,

> Sometimes, and it was a directive from supervisors, that a couple of pieces from … the next day's paper would be scheduled to go live [on the website] … so that the paper the people were getting that day didn't feel stale … the idea was that if someone saw something in the paper that they want to share, they'll be able to find it [on the website].

In this passage, an interesting aspect of Sarah's text-processing work emerges. We can see here that her work happens in a sort of cycle that is closely related to how news texts move on social media. Sarah not only refers to Facebook to gauge what stories are worth placing on the Urban News homepage, her supervisors also foreground the lead stories from the print version of the paper on the website's homepage in order to facilitate readers sharing the articles on Facebook. This sequence calls attention to the predominant role of text-processing activities in contemporary newswork.

The Social Organization of Newswork

Alex's and Sarah's accounts of their everyday work show some of the ways that activities to produce, process, and modify texts are a central feature of today's newswork. In this section I illustrate how this type of writing for digital news is coordinated by a management strategy for news production referred to as convergence journalism. I devote particular attention to how the social relations of convergence journalism hook reporters' work into organizational processes of commercialization and generalist reporting. Surfacing the ways that commercialization and generalist reporting shape newswork clarifies how convergence journalism coordinates the standard genre of salacious, sensational crime stories about HIV criminalization.

Critical social science that analyzes the content of news coverage of HIV criminalization often understands the source of problematic discourse to be tied to historically rooted racist news discourse (Lupton 1999; McKay et al. 2011; J. Miller 2005) and structural racism (Persson and Newman 2008). In this section of the chapter, I want to show how a study of social organization can contribute to understandings of how problematic news coverage of HIV non-disclosure cases is produced. Here, I build on the work of critical scholars who call attention to the long history of stigmatizing news reports of HIV criminalization by showing that the social conditions of convergence journalism make it exceedingly difficult to disrupt the genre of crime reporting in which these stigmatizing discourses proliferate. This is because convergence journalism creates conditions in which the work of creating news is about processing existing texts into multiple formats as quickly as possible, and with very limited opportunity for original journalistic investigation. Furthermore, the source texts that reporters are left to rely on often emphasize the sort of sensational, superficial tropes that have defined news reports about HIV criminalization for decades.

The Commercialization of Digital News

Since the invention of the printing press, a central concern around journalism has been the conflict between the public interest and the self-interest of those who control news production (McManus 2019). For almost two centuries, media moguls have provided news as mass commodity – a type of news that John McManus (2019) describes as "a cheap, popular kind of journalism designed more to turn than fill heads." This tension between profit and quality journalism lies at the heart of discussions about the commercialization of news. The commercialization of news can refer to "any action intended to boost profit that interferes with a journalist's or news organization's best effort to maximize public understanding of those issues and events that shape the community they claim to serve" (McManus 2008, 219). While the demands of the market have always clashed with the production of quality journalism in complex ways, the highly precarious economic circumstances in which online news is produced today push news agencies to operate with great concern for the commercial viability of their product

One of the primary ways that news organizations have transformed their news production practices in order to protect their profit margins is by prioritizing multimedia reporting that is intended for online, digital platforms. As news organizations restructure themselves to contend with a hyper-competitive and economically uncertain media landscape, digital news production provides a cost-effective strategy for producing low-cost and widely spreadable news content (Bakker 2012; Saridou, Lia-Paschalia, and Veglis 2017, 1006). The journalists I interviewed regularly explained that their news agencies have restructured their organization to steadily prioritize the production of digital, online news over other platforms. For example, when I interviewed Shawn he had worked as a full-time reporter at a major Canadian newspaper for four years. Even over that rather short period of time, he recognizes that the newsroom has become "a lot more integrated. It used to be a web desk and a print desk. Now it's a lot more, they came out and said, 'we're a digital organization that happens to print a newspaper,' trying to make print an afterthought rather than the first thing they think about."

This sort of "digital first" approach to news production that Shawn describes shapes the everyday newswork of Alex and Sarah. One way that the commercialization of digital news coordinates their activities is by intensifying the pace of their newswork. To keep step with the frenzied pace of digital news production, Alex and Sarah lean on quick and efficient text-production and processing activities. For example, Alex's account of his hurried workday shows how he repurposes and spreads a common text, such as an interview, to supply content to multiple platforms on an hourly basis. Sarah, who worked in a setting at which Alex's text might arrive, continuously processes texts into online news to keep the news agency's homepage "fresh" – an activity that she would repeat at least twenty-five times throughout her shift.

The relations of commercialization also coordinate the content of texts that reporters generate. Both Alex and Sarah described how their work practices are shaped by their understanding of what sort of news story will attract a high volume of readers online. For instance, Alex explained that he models his writing on news stories that, according to data that his editors circulate, are viewed, liked, and shared online most often. Meanwhile, Sarah described how her editorial decisions are based on evaluating the popularity of news stories on other news websites and social media platforms. This type of newswork that Alex and Sarah do to produce news texts that masses of online readers will consume is a central part of their work practices within the business model of convergence journalism. For decades, newspapers relied heavily on audience and advertisers to generate revenue. Today, as readers' print subscriptions and revenues from print advertisements wane dramatically, digital data that quantifies how online visitors view, click, "like," and share an online news story is vital to news organizations, as this data is monetized by attracting advertisers to news sites (Benbunan-Fich and Fich 2004; Hanusch and Edson Tandoc 2019; Napoli 2010; Vu 2014).

Journalists and scholars of journalism have a range of perspectives on how these types of digital metrics shape newswork. As Angele Christin writes in her book *Metrics at Work: Journalism and the Contested Meaning of Algorithms*, "coverage of algorithms and digital metrics [in newsrooms] has split between technological utopianism and dire warnings" (2020, 3). While optimists promote digital metrics as a way "to make more informed, efficient, and objective decisions" (3), less hopeful researchers and practitioners have expressed serious concerns about how the commercialization of digital news constrains reporters' work and threatens the quality of journalism.

A specific point of unease has to do with working conditions that set reporters up to produce "click bait" news texts as quickly as possible and with an eye towards the news texts' popularity online. As the argument goes, news production practices that are geared towards rapidly producing widely read articles favour the publication of simple, uncontentious, and easy-to-obtain news stories, as opposed to long-form, nuanced, and more expensive journalistic endeavours (Christin 2020, 2; Davies 2008; Karlsson 2011; Saridou, Lia-Paschalia, and Veglis 2017, 1009). One can recognize, for instance, that the constant speed at which Alex is expected to produce news texts, and the pace at which Sarah is supposed to process and "refresh" news texts, limit opportunities to assess or reflect on the quality of news content. The threats that the commercialization of digital news poses to journalistic integrity and ethics were impressed upon me during an interview I conducted with a veteran reporter named Lisa. Lisa has worked at News Centre (the same news agency as Alex) for over 20 years. She described her concerns about the pace of online news:

> Stories have a shelf-life of not even a day, or a day and it's over, people have lost interest. So, whether it ended up being true or false or misrepresented by us, or just a complete misrepresentation of any context to do with what's happening, can be completely irrelevant … because now we're on to a story about, you know, whatever the next thing is.

What this passage starts to show is that while convergence may serve as a strategy for "efficient" news production, and a way for news organizations to commercialize their product in response to the uncertain economic conditions that they face, it is also an approach that raises doubts around journalistic integrity and robust reporting. It is difficult to conceptualize how reporters could possibly consistently produce nuanced and complex accounts of issues within newsrooms that hook their work into the rapid pace of online, digital news production. Lisa also grappled with how to square her understanding of the principles of journalism with the organizational demand for reporters to produce news content that will be read and shared widely online. She explained:

> We're constantly being told with our online stories which ones are the most popular. But also . . . you can write two headlines for your story and the [software] system will push them out there, and then you can see which headline is attracting more clicks so that at a certain point you can just bail on the more boring headline and go to the salacious headline that's working better … I think it's the whole idea of news judgment. Are you trying to shape or broaden or strengthen democracy or just sell people something? That's the worry, I guess.

In this segment Lisa helps to surface how processes of commercialization coordinate newswork that contribute to the production and reproduction of the standard genre of sensational crime story about HIV criminalization. Headlines understood to be "working better" are those that draw the highest volume of readers to the story, often, as Lisa suggests, by being shocking or provocative in tone. In the case of HIV and the criminal law, headlines that alert readers to dangerous, threatening, hyper-sexualized outsiders are more likely to grab readers' attention than those that treat the issue as a complex and nuanced public health issue. As long as news organizations rely on web traffic as one of their main strategies for attracting advertising revenues, this pattern of salacious reporting on HIV criminalization is likely to continue.

Generalist Reporting

Along with the commercialization of digital news, a second relation of convergence journalism that shapes reporters' everyday newswork is the trend towards generalist reporting. Convergence management structures often position reporters in news organizations as "generalists." One of the easiest ways for news publishers to save money is to do away with the beat structure, in which a reporter specializes in a particular news topic, and instead pay one reporter (often young journalists) as a generalist reporter to do several jobs (Coxon 2013; Van Leuven, Vanhaelewyn, and Raeymaeckers 2021). Within converged newsrooms, generalist reporters are expected to be flexible and adaptable in terms of the topics that they report on and to be proficient at multi-skilling. Generalist reporters regularly carry out multiple tasks at once and combine distinct news-gathering and story-telling techniques that were once separate in analogue environments. The shift towards generalist reporting in converged news agencies alters traditional newsroom structures, operations, and divisions of labour (Chadha and Wells 2016; Mitchelstein and Boczkowski 2009).

The social relations of generalist reporting inform how the reporters I spoke to understand their everyday work. For example, Alex explained that in his newsroom,

> You're a bit of a generalist, yeah. And as you go along you can sort of develop more of a specific beat. But I mean, our newsroom ... is sort of changing ... I think they're wanting to get rid of beats, like we lost our sports reporter and they're not replacing him with a sports reporter they're replacing him by a generalist reporter, we lost our arts reporter and they're not replacing him with an arts reporter they're replacing him with a generalist reporter as well. So, I don't know. I don't know how I feel about that.

One of the most notable aspects of Alex's newswork as a generalist is the wide variety of news topics he covers. The news stories he produces span diverse topics such as business, public health, education, and francophone affairs. Alex is also a multi-skilled reporter. His description of his everyday newswork details how he utilizes various digital technologies to source, construct, and disseminate news in both French and English. As news agencies cut spending on specialist reporters and employ fewer generalist reporters, those, like Alex, who remain in the newsroom are required to do more (produce more content, more often, across more platforms, about more topics) with less (time, resources, and space to do in-depth reporting on a specific topic). In order to continuously produce news content on a range of topics across multiple news platforms, Alex's writing for digital news is focused on repurposing and transferring a common source text to multiple sites within his news agency.

The trend towards generalist reporting shaped Sarah's everyday text-based work as a web editor as well. She explained that due to staff layoffs at her news organization, the scope of her newswork expanded considerably. Sarah described that she edited the homepage

> for all markets across Canada, so nine cities … we were a really small team, so we're running nine different homepages for all the different cities and on any given day, because there were a few layoffs, there were only two of us running the site. So how it would kind of end up working towards the end is that there was one person whose job was to do the homepages, and the other person was just feeding in that content, editing, and putting the stories up

This passage helps to show how Sarah's work comes to centre on activities that consist of processing texts as quickly and efficiently as possible. The laying-off of editors who might specialize in a particular geographic region means that Sarah and her remaining colleagues are left to find ways to edit the homepages for nine different websites simultaneously. In such a context, the editorial practices that Sarah has time to complete are reduced to, as she described, "copy and pasting it pretty much," and she devoted less time to fact-checking or more in-depth editing work.

Journalism scholars have expressed concerns about how this demand for flexible, multi-skilled, generalist reporting within converged newsrooms blurs the distinction between technicians and journalists and also has the potential to distract journalists from their primary task of news gathering and coverage (Chadha and Wells 2016, 2). I came to understand how these types of concerns about generalist reporting practices materialize in the content of news stories about HIV criminalization during an interview I conducted with a reporter named Allen.

Allen has worked at a newspaper, which I will refer to as the *Pine City Guardian*, for over thirty-five years. Much of the paper's content focuses on local issues, but it also includes syndicated national and international news content from news agencies that are owned by the same media corporation. Over Allen's tenure with the *Pine City Guardian*, the field of journalism and his work setting have undergone profound changes. Allen has an extensive background and training as a photographer, and for most of his career at the *Pine City Guardian*, he worked exclusively as a photo-journalist. Recently, however, Allen has had to confront an increasing pressure to be a flexible, multi-skilled, generalist reporter who produces news content about diverse news topics across a number of news platforms. As Allen describes,

> I had a nice portfolio in 1982 at the *Pine City Guardian*. Pretty much stuck to just photography for I'd say twenty years until I started getting into a little bit of writing, just writing simple stories to go with my photos and then over the last number of years, because of the decrease in reporters, it seems like everyone became multimedia journalists, which we call ourselves now. So, there are trained reporters who learn how to take pictures and trained photographers who learn how to write stories, so we kind of mix together and cover as much as we can. I'd say for at least the last ten years I guess I've been doing, now I do more writing than photography.

The social relations of convergence journalism echo throughout Allen's description of his newswork. Allen understands his transition from working exclusively as a photographer to taking on the role of a "multimedia journalist" to be tied to the restructuring of his news organization. As his organization reduces resource spending and employs fewer reporters, Allen is expected to be a multi-skilled generalist reporter.

Allen's position as a generalist, multimedia journalist means that he covers diverse news topics. Occasionally this includes covering stories about crime and the Canadian correctional system. A notable case that Allen reported involved a thirty-year-old male, who I will call Lewis, who was convicted on multiple counts of aggravated sexual assault for not disclosing his HIV-positive status to sexual partners. He was sentenced to twenty years in prison. The charges against Lewis were laid in Elm Town. Allen reported on the man's parole hearings that took place in 2013, 2015, and 2016 in five news articles that ran in the *Pine City Guardian* and the *Elm Town Chronicle*.

Allen's news articles about the parole hearings display some of the common, troubling features of mainstream news coverage of HIV criminalization that I identified at the outset of this chapter. For one, his reporting takes place in what we've referred to as "criminal justice time" in which news coverage of criminal HIV non-disclosure cases is sequenced upon the standard criminal legal processing of a case. For example, Allen's reporting only brings Lewis and the issue of HIV criminalization into public discourse at moments when the case proceeds through a standard stage of the criminal justice process – a parole hearing. Allen's coverage of the parole hearings also works to produce HIV criminalization as a straightforward crime story by relying heavily on language associated with the criminal legal system. Each of his stories about a parole hearing follows a similar structure: (1) the story begins by affirming Lewis's status as a "notorious sex offender" or "convicted sex offender"; (2) the charges that Lewis faces are restated; (3) a description of the most recent parole hearing follows; and (4) the article concludes by listing the next steps in the criminal-legal system processing of his case. This style of reporting not only produces HIV non-disclosure as a crime story, it also objectifies Lewis as a criminal subject. Examining the everyday newswork practices that generate this sort of news coverage, and the social worlds in which they occur, reveals how the institutional relations of convergence journalism produce and reproduce the sensational genre of crime stories about HIV criminalization.

As a generalist reporter, Allen meets the demand to quickly and efficiently produce news content on a range of news topics largely by processing texts produced by expert authorities. For example, he explained that his work covering crime stories commonly begins by scanning police press releases to identify relevant stories to pursue:

> With the police, I just usually do the stuff they send out, they send a daily update of what's happening on their side, the police side, and usually I take a look at that and re-write those. I check, the police has a portal that I go to that's for the media that has all their releases, I just look for ones that are in this area ... they write a very dry thing and I go through it and I try to, not jazz it up, but make it a little more readable for the newspaper.

I look more closely at how reporters' work hooks into police communications work in the next chapter. For now, I want to foreground that Allen's work to identify news stories is based largely in locating readily available, online, digital sources. Allen's newswork process is mostly hooked into easily accessible texts from criminal legal authorities because the social conditions of convergence journalism limit opportunities to conduct further research or to consider multiple sources.

Allen's work practices to base his newswork upon readily accessible digital texts make sense in the converged structure that he works in as a generalist reporter. These desk-top activities make it possible for him to meet an organizational demand to cover diverse news topics and to use multiple story-telling techniques. For example, when I asked Allen about how he selects textual information upon which to base news stories he replied: "pretty much I'll use everything they [the police] send me, that the editor decides on."

Allen's work to process texts, such as police press releases, is noteworthy because it brings into view the sort of talk and text that are most readily available to reporters whose work practices are organized by the relations of convergence journalism. One can imagine that Allen could have based his reporting on a different type of source text, a report produced by a community-based HIV advocacy organization, for instance. However, Allen's work practices mainly depend on texts that are produced by criminal legal authorities and function to maintain a status quo, as opposed to texts from community-based HIV activist groups or legal advocates that introduce critiques of HIV criminalization or put forward counter discourses. This structure calls to mind Stuart Hall's observations about how those in powerful institutional positions have privileged access to the press. Allen's experiences show that this structure makes it challenging for reporters to resist reproducing longstanding societal views of people living with HIV and criminality and help to explain the reproduction of stigmatizing, objectifying discourses within news coverage of HIV criminalization.

Institutional Ethnography and the Study of Overlapping Ruling Relations

So far, reporters' descriptions of their everyday newswork in this chapter help us to understand the scope of their newswork practices to produce digital news content. We tend not to consider the types of quick text-processing work that reporters spoke about as we scroll through streams of online news stories. The attention-grabbing headlines, punchy quotations, and consistent updates on the surface of digital news texts obscure the steps journalists take to create these reports. However, when we read reporters' accounts of their work for social organization we can recognize how the corporate media management strategy of convergence journalism pulls their work into processes of commercialization and generalist reporting. And so, on one hand, this IE offers a vantage point for understanding what it looks like to write for digital news and, in particular, how a standard genre of crime stories about HIV criminalization takes form.

At the same time, the interviews in this chapter present an opportunity to reflect on the scope of IE as an approach to critical social inquiry. As is common for IE, this analysis starts with interviews that focus on participants' everyday work practices and projects analysis beyond the local site to show their activities are embedded in trans-local ruling relations. Readers will recognize that the concept of ruling relations is central to IE. Dorothy Smith (2005, 10) understands ruling relations to be

> that extraordinary yet ordinary complex of relations that are textually mediated, that connect us across space and time and organize our everyday lives – the corporations, government bureaucracies, academic and professional discourses, mass media, and the complex of relations that connect them.

Elsewhere, Smith (2002, 45) adds that ruling relations

> coordinate people's activities across and beyond local sites of everyday experience. We know them variously as bureaucracy, discourse (in the Foucauldian sense), management, mass media, institutions, and so on and so on ... they are extra- or trans-local and based in texts of various kinds (print, computer, film, television, and so on). Such concepts as information, knowledge, "culture," science, and the like are rethought as relations among people that rely on materiality of the text and its increasingly complex technologies. Institutions are specific functional foci within the complex of ruling relations.

It is important to notice that Smith's concept of ruling relations relies on the notion of institutions and that institutions are defined as functional complexes. Institutions, such as education, law, and health care, are distinguished from one another on the basis of the function that they perform. Thus, fixing my ethnographic gaze and analytic focus on the newsroom helps to illuminate how the institution of news media is coordinated from several different organizational levels, including news organization business management, news editors, fellow reporters, website technicians, camera operators, radio and television producers, and more. Some institutional ethnographies might focus analysis within the bounds of the newsroom. Such an IE that traces the ruling relations within news media organizations would be useful for understanding the social architecture of digital-first newsrooms and could, for example, be applied to identify the structures that facilitate or hinder efficient news production. At the same time a close reading of reporters' accounts of their routine newswork in this chapter starts to reveal that their work is also intricately tied to work that others are doing in sites beyond the walls of their news corporation. We can see, for example, that throughout reporters' workdays they process a litany of texts that arrive at their desks from other institutions. I was particularly struck by the extent to which reporters work with one type of text in particular: police press releases. For example, recall the way that Allen's newswork activities are primarily hooked into texts that police produce.

Recognizing that reporters' work is not only intricately tied to work that is happening in other sectors of the newsroom but also relies on work that is taking place in the realm of policing invites questions about the scope of institutional ethnographic studies of ruling relations. For instance, we might ask: Is institutional ethnographic research limited to investigating ruling relations within a particular institution (such as news production)? Can IE accommodate an analysis across different institutions? Throughout this book I want to suggest that IE can be used to examine the intersection of multiple functional complexes. The spirit of IE analysis positions the researcher to show how different institutions overlap and intersect with one another. Smith (1987, 160) suggests that "we might imagine institutions as nodes or knots in the [ruling] relations ... coordinating multiple strands of action into a functional complex." If we extend Smith's metaphor of nodes and knots to consider relations not only within an individual functional complex but across them, we have a route into promoting IE research that surfaces how different institutions are related with one another.

While there is a lineage of influential and generative IE research that focuses on the social relations within a specific functional complex, scholars have also pushed institutional ethnographers to show how different institutional complexes are connected with one another. As Viviane Namaste writes:

> analysis that restricts itself to one institution can be limited to the extent that it does not understand the links or the lack of connection among different institutions, as well as the attending consequences for the institutional ordering of experience. (Namaste 2006, 167)

In focusing on connections between institutions, Namaste (2006, 170–1) resists a sort of individualizing quality of the standard conception of social relations in IE. Namaste's study of how transgender people navigate the bureaucratic process of changing one's legal identity on government documents moves beyond an analysis of a single institution and shows how the process of attaining government documents is lived through a variety of institutions, such as gender identity clinics, health care, and immigration systems. Namaste underlines, "given this ... practitioners of institutional ethnography ought to devote some attention to the development of methodologies that allow us to under-stand the relations between different institutions."

In the next chapters of this book, instead of producing an account that concentrates exclusively on the organizational and institutional practices of news production, I attempt to formulate a mode of criti-cal inquiry that shows trans-local ruling relations by empirically investigating multiple institutions. As an institutional ethnographer, this means not only reading interview transcripts to uncover "what people say about the work they do that connects them to the work others are doing elsewhere and elsewhen" (Abu-Lughod et al. 2002, 31) but actually going to and investigating the work that other people do elsewhere within a range of institutional sites. I related to tran-scripts of interviews with journalists as directions for where to go and who to talk to next. Throughout the rest of this book, this leads me to interview police communications officers to learn about policing, HIV legal experts to learn about the criminal law, and service providers at AIDS service organizations to learn about support services for peo-ple living with HIV. Investigating this range of work activities in this range of institutional settings helps bring into view an entire complex of activities that both produce and contest the standard crime genre news story about HIV criminalization.

In the next chapter, I focus on how reporters' newswork is coordi-nated with the work of police communications units that publish press releases. I turn my attention to that empirical site because reporters almost always named police news releases as their source for crime genre stories about HIV criminalization and because news stories that are based on police press releases are a notorious source of critique among community-based HIV advocates. These types of crime stories are viewed as particularly stigmatizing and are therefore deserving of closer attention. Understanding how the coordination of newswork and police work produces stigmatizing crime genre stories about HIV criminalization also helps to underscore the importance of seeing how social relations cut across multiple institutions.

Chapter Three

The Coordination of Police Work and Newswork

The previous chapter can be understood as an invitation for readers to contemplate the news in ways that are not typically available in studies of news content and representation. I wanted to bring readers into the newsroom, and to make the social world of news production visible by illuminating the everyday work that reporters do to research, develop, write, and circulate news stories. Reporters' accounts illuminated that the conditions of newswork in convergence journalism are likely to produce sensational accounts of topics such as HIV criminalization because they set reporters up to rely on existing texts that emphasize sensational and superficial aspects of HIV non-disclosure cases. As reporters I spoke with described their newswork they regularly characterized police news releases as particularly influential source texts that made it possible to produce news stories about HIV criminal non-disclosure cases.

In this chapter I concentrate on the production of news stories that are based on police press releases because these stories inaugurate criminal justice time reporting and are the first reports to emerge in what often becomes a trajectory of coverage of a given case. Furthermore, this genre of news story has been a real concern among HIV activists. Advocacy organizations I work with are the most alarmed when someone's mugshot from a police news release appears in a major daily news publication and when articles about alleged HIV non-disclosures are produced as short, decontextualized crime stories. These are the stories that we try to respond to quickly through letters to the editor or direct messages to journalists that underline the variety of harms these articles pose to people living with HIV and LGBTQ2S+ groups, and ask journalists to refrain from publishing the names and images of individuals charged with not disclosing their HIV-positive status (Bell 2017; Kirkup 2014–15; O'Byrne 2011).

My central argument in this chapter is that the professional worlds of police communications and journalism are brought into close relationship with one another through reporters' work with police news releases. As reporters strategically select parts of police news releases and recontextualize them as news, they accommodate the flow of police information and reasoning into the mainstream press.[1] This allows the police's formulation of crime, danger, risk, and security to be active in mainstream news discourse that flows into people's everyday lives.

My empirical account of the coordination of newswork and police communications work is organized into four sections. First, I display an example of a police news release and show how a reporter transfers the text into a news article. Reporters' descriptions of their work settings in this first section start to suggest reasons that police texts are such a common source of news stories in contemporary newsrooms. In the second section of this chapter, "Radio Silence and Terse Cop Speak," I draw on interviews with reporters to show how police texts enter into their everyday newswork routines and describe particular ways that reporters activate these texts. The third section, "Those Are Our Facts," is an account of the work that police corporate communications departments do to produce texts that distribute information to news organizations. My interview with a police professional named David, who works in a police corporate communications department, helps to show how newswork practices and police work practices are brought together through shared understandings of the facts of a case, and constructions of risk and public safety. Finally, in the fourth section, I reflect on the implications that the coordination of police communications work and

---

1 While reporters' work with police press releases pulls the social relations of police communications into news production processes, it is also important to recognize that when a reporter activates a police press release, they are being pulled into the relations of policing. This can occur as a news reader reads an article that circulates a police news release and then comes forward to police as a potential victim or with information about the person accused of a crime.

It is challenging to identify terminology that accurately describes the relationship and many directions of flow between reporters' work practices and work that happens in police communications departments. Often, institutional ethnographers will describe that one's work is "hooked into," "geared into," "entered into," or "pulled into" the social relations of work done in other sites. However, this language can suggest a unidirectional relationship between the work that is done in one site and the work done in other sites. In an effort to build a more relational approach to studying the relationship between the work done in newsrooms and police communications departments, I have used phrasing such as "coordinated with" and "connected to" throughout this chapter.

newswork has on public knowledge of HIV criminalization and common understandings of powerful concepts such as public health, risk, safety, and security. Before I present reporters' accounts of their work with police news releases, I provide some context for the work of police communications departments and outline the approach to text analysis that I employ throughout this chapter.

Police Communications Units and Police News Releases

Criminal justice scholars have acknowledged that studies of policing often overlook the great deal of work that police forces do to control information and to manage their image. In this chapter, I add to studies that call attention to forms of police work that centre on patrolling facts and reproducing the symbolic order and legitimacy of police (Chermak 1995; Ericson, Baranek, and Chan 1989, 1991). From the very outset of the modern policing apparatus, policing work has been accomplished in part through media technologies that allow the force to "police at a distance" (Reeves and Packer 2013, 360). Since the 1770s, police forces have distributed texts such as mug shots, "wanted posters," printed newspapers, handbills, and professional police gazettes to broadly communicate crimes, stolen goods, and potential threats (Reeves and Packer 2013, 364). These practices allowed police to extend the reach of their surveillance while remaining relatively inconspicuous (370). As Reeves and Packer describe, "police media were used to publicize suspects' identities, diffusing police responsibilities to the public and deterring crime through the insecurity of categorical suspicion and ubiquitous surveillance" (369). That is to say, the press's reliance on police sources is not a new phenomenon. Since the analogue era, police public relations departments have been adept at ensuring that their texts flow into reporters' work settings (Ericson, Baranek, and Chan 1989; Reeves and Packer 2013). However, as the continuous cycle of digital news production has intensified the scope and pace of reporters' work, journalists have come to rely extensively on such digital public relations texts as sources of news (Davies 2008; Lewis, Williams, and Franklin 2008; Winters et al. 2019).

Historical analyses of police communications and public relations departments in the United States situate them as responses to public outcries about violent police tactics utilized during the civil rights protests of the 1960s (Motschall and Cao 2002, 154). It was during this period that police departments established press offices or public information units to facilitate their interactions with mainstream media (154). Over the years, police public relations work developed into a more formalized and professionalized part of police organizations. Police forces began to recruit professional communications experts and shifted away from reacting and responding to media requests and towards more proactive communications activities (Mawby 1999, 272).

Today, units within police departments that were once commonly referred to as the "Press Office" or "Press and Public Relations" are most often called "Corporate Communications" departments. Criminologist Tom Mawby (2010) suggests that "the use of the name 'corporate communications' is not simply re-labelling; it denotes the strategic direction in which police communications is moving and supported by an increase in communications budgets and the size of departments" (129). This means that police forces are committing greater resources to their public relations and communication activities at a time when media organizations are reducing their news-gathering resources (Cheng 2021), thus raising important questions about contemporary news organizations' capacity to report on policing issues and, ultimately, to hold the police to account (131).

Police press releases are a central part of how HIV non-disclosure is policed. Police forces regularly publish the name, image, and other personal information of an individual facing criminal charges related to alleged HIV non-disclosure to attract attention to these cases with a view to strengthening the charges they are making. Police press releases about HIV non-disclosure cases enlist the public in policing activities, for example, by trying to identify further complainants and encouraging people to come forward to police with information that they may have about the individual facing charges. Some reporters I spoke with subscribe to police listservs and have news releases emailed to their inbox regularly. Other reporters explained that they scan police forces' social media sites for URL links to news releases. Digital police news release texts feature bold, eye-catching headings that typically include the brand markings (such as the police department's name, logo, and slogan) of the police force issuing the news release. The heading also expresses the alleged criminal offence as an alert, for example, a "sexual assault alert." In addition, news releases list phone numbers that one can call to provide police investigators with information, the police division that is responsible for the case (sex crimes, for example), the name of the detective constable overseeing the case, and the case number.

It is important to specify that in this chapter I am focusing on just one moment in the potential sequence of news stories about criminal HIV non-disclosure cases – the point at which criminal charges are laid (this is also the stage at which police press releases are issued). Sometimes, when criminal charges are laid, HIV non-disclosure cases are covered in a single, brief news story based on details included in a news release. However, in other instances, when a criminal HIV non-disclosure case goes to trial, there is a subsequent trajectory of news stories that may include forms of journalism that rely less on police texts. For example, in high-profile criminal HIV non-disclosure cases, journalists may attend the trial and conduct interviews in order to produce first-hand accounts of the court proceedings. The initial news stories that are the focus of this chapter often set the tone for subsequent reporting about criminal HIV non-disclosure cases.

A key feature of Studies in the Social Organization of Knowledge (SSOK) is a close attention to the central role that texts play in coordinating ruling relations (D.E. Smith 1993). Texts, such as police press releases that journalists activate and produce in their work processes, make it possible for the same set of words, numbers, or images to appear in multiple local sites. In so doing they standardize, regulate, and authorize people's activities (D.E. Smith 2001, 160). Dorothy Smith understands texts as "key devices in hooking people's activities in particular local settings and at particular times into the transcending organizations of ruling relations" (164). Thus, for Smith, it is not enough to study police press releases as sources of information about police forces. Rather, these texts must be studied ethnographically "as they enter into people's local practice of writing, drawing, reading, looking and so on. They must be examined as they co-ordinate people's activities" (160). As an institutional ethnographer, I treat police news releases as texts that bridge the local sites of reporters' everyday embodied activities and trans-local, abstracted ruling relations (Weir and Mykhalovskiy 2010, 22). Conceptualizing police news release texts as coordinators of ruling relations makes it possible to illuminate the ways that reporters are entered into ongoing social relations when they work with these documents (D.E. Smith 1993, 6). Such an approach to sociological inquiry offers a strategy for making visible how the activities of journalists are connected to other forms of ruling that shape the experiences of criminalized groups, including people who live with HIV in Canada.

Studies of Recontextualization and Professional Writing Practices

My institutional ethnographic study of how police press releases operate as texts that coordinate ruling relations is informed by analyses of recontexualization. Broadly, accounts of recontexualization call attention to how parts of discourse from one context are selected and used as resources in creating new meaning in a different context (Koskela 2010; Solin 2004). Per Linell (1998) defines recontextualization as

the dynamic transfer-and-transformation of something from one dis-
course/text-in-context … to another. Recontextualization involves the
extrication of some part or aspect from a text or discourse, or from a genre
of texts of discourses, and the fitting of this part or aspect into another
context, i.e., another text or discourse and its use and environment. (Linell
1998, 145)

Studying texts with an eye to recontextualization can direct analytic
attention to how social organization is accomplished across professional
boundaries. Linell (1998, 150) suggests that when labellings, problem
definitions, and biographical fragments of people are recontextualized,
"we can observe a mixing, blending, or blurring of different voices and
interests in the discourse of particular categories of professionals, in
specific genres of discourses or within particular texts. Elements from
different discourses and discourse types often partly merge, partly stay
on to compete with each other." Analyses of recontextualization provide a vantage point to observe how professionals strategically select,
endorse, edit, subdue, or silence parts or aspects of discourses when
information is recontextualized from one professional's perspective to
another's (150–1) (Solin 2004, 271).

I've found that thinking about recontextualization has been helpful
for my understanding of how professional writing practices connect the
realms of police communications and journalism and for conceptualizing how these coordinated work activities reproduce the ruling relations
of HIV criminalization. Other institutional ethnographers have noticed
that HIV criminalization is partly sustained through the work that people do to transfer texts across professional boundaries. For example,
Chris Sanders's (2015) ethnographic study of HIV criminalization looks
closely at public health nurses' documentary styles. His research shows
how a record produced in a public health counselling setting comes to
be written in ways that are intended for readers who work in criminal justice settings. His account displays how nurses' documentary
practices and styles are designed to either accommodate or disrupt the
flow of information from case files to criminal trial proceedings. Elsewhere, Eric Mykhalovskiy has shown that an important feature of the
social organization of HIV criminalization is the intersection of public
health and criminal law regulation. The context of HIV criminalization
includes "the movement of public health knowledge into court proceedings where it is recontextualized and comes to coordinate relations
of criminal law decision making and punishment" (Mykhalovskiy 2011,
674). This trajectory of institutional ethnographic research that attends
to processes of recontextualization brings into view the centrality of

textual practices in large-scale forms of organization that occur across professional boundaries (Mykhalovskiy 2003, 336; Sanders 2015, 401). I try and add to that line of research here by illuminating the various work activities that facilitate the flow of police information and forms of reasoning about HIV criminalization to the everyday worlds of news readers.

Police Texts as News Texts

In the first section of this chapter, I want show how the social conditions of contemporary news organizations, as described in the previous chapter, structure reporters' dependence on police news releases. As a starting point for an institutional ethnographic study of how reporters work with police news releases, consider the following texts that I found during fieldwork. The first text is a short news report with the headline "Man, 27, Charged after Failing to Tell Sexual Partners about HIV Status." The news article publicizes the man's name, age, photo, HIV-positive status, the date at which he was diagnosed with HIV, and details the criminal charges that he faces. The article also describes how he met his sex partners, identifies their gender, age, and their alleged HIV-positive status.

A close reading of the news article starts to direct attention to ways that reporters rely on text and talk from police communications departments in order to produce accounts of crime. For example, while the topic of the news report is the man facing criminal charges, it is telling that the subject of almost half of the sentences is the police: "police have arrested," "police said," "police have charged." The reporter's work with the police press release effectively translates the text that police published to build a case against this individual into a news story about what police have said and the actions that police have carried out.

The extent to which the police mediate messages about the arrest that circulate in the press comes into view even more clearly when one pairs the news text with the news release that Toronto Police Services published about the case on their Facebook page. The press release is headed by the Toronto Police Service logo and slogan "To Serve and Protect." Under the headline is script that reads: "Sexual Assault Alert, [the person's name], 27 [the person's age], Additional Charges Laid, Police Concerned There May Be More Victims." The mugshot photo of the person facing charges takes up the bulk of the space in the press release, and under the image, phone numbers to contact investigators and Crime Stoppers are included. As one reads the details the police have included in the press release, one finds that significant portions of the news release text have been transferred into the news article verbatim. In fact, the news article introduces no new information, details, or context to add to what was included in the police news release. In this instance, the reporter's work to produce the news article consisted of simply copying the text that police published and recontextualizing it as a news article.

One reporter, named Leah, who covers breaking news understands news articles that rest heavily on police texts as an unfortunate, but inevitable part of newswork in the context of contemporary newsrooms:

> You'll see arrest stories that are really straightforward, just written from press releases, those kinds of stories are really easy to do. In an ideal world, you would never just write from a press release and let it stop there, you would always want to go out and talk to people in community and talk to people involved, you would want to have context and all that stuff, but the reality is that doesn't always happen.

What Leah's account starts to show is that the working conditions of news production limit reporters' capacity to produce news stories with contextual depth or that incorporate diverse voices and perspectives beyond the police texts that are readily available to reporters. Leah explained that, as a journalist, she would prefer to dig deeper than police news releases as sources for news stories, but news organizations' demand for constant news content sets up reporters to engage in work practices that will produce news articles as quickly as possible. As she described:

> It's someone's job to write those quick [crime] stories and get them out there. Often those people writing those stories are young and inexperienced or just may not have thought of it. Like I just think about when I started doing this, I didn't know all of the stuff that I know now. Now when I'm reporting on something I'll go, okay I remember this, this, and this case, I know the history of this, so I can put something into context or I can challenge something and say, no, that's not how that normally happens. All of that stuff, people writing those stories probably haven't thought about, what are the ramifications of this story? What has the Supreme Court said about this? How does this all fit together? They're just writing like five-inch "police have arrested so and so and want people to know such and such." There's no thought that goes into it. It's like content generation.

In this segment, Leah underlines how the two relations of convergence journalism that became clear in the previous chapter structure the newswork of reporters who cover crime and breaking news. First, her account indicates that the work practices of reporters who cover crime and breaking news are geared to processes of commercialization. The reporter's "job to write those quick stories and get them out there" meets an institutional demand for a consistent stream of news content generation that will attract online news consumers.

The second relation of convergence journalism that is visible in Leah's account has to do with generalist reporting. Leah describes the particular challenges that arise when generalist reporters who lack experience and expertise covering complex criminal legal issues report on crime stories: important historical and legal contexts fall away, and reporters end up relying on texts that police produce in order to generate news content. Leah's account of reporters' work with police news releases is valuable, because it shows how the structure of news organizations position reporters to lean on police documents in order to do their job. However, as I interviewed reporters who had worked with police news releases to produce news stories about HIV criminalization, I started to notice ways that journalists' newswork is coordinated with social relations that extend outside of the newsroom as well.

Radio Silence and Terse Cop Speak: Reporters' Work with Police Press Releases

I started to recognize ways that reporters' newswork is connected to police communications work during an interview with a reporter named Laura who works at the *Daily Gazette*. I reached out to Laura to request an interview in the days after a news story she wrote about a man who faced criminal charges for allegedly not disclosing his HIV-positive status to sex partners circulated online. I wanted to talk with Laura to gain a better sense of how she came to cover this story and to know more about the steps she took to develop the article. At the time I interviewed Laura, she was working as a summer intern at the *Daily Gazette* while she completed her journalism degree. Most of her daily work as an intern consisted of monitoring and covering breaking news stories over an eight-hour shift. Laura typically worked from 8:00 a.m. until 4:00 p.m. and occasionally from 4:00 p.m. until midnight. She was unexpectedly called to work an overnight shift from midnight to 8:00 a.m. the night before our interview. She generously met me at 10:00 a.m. anyway, even though her shift ended only a couple of hours before.

Laura's account of her newswork was fundamental for my understanding of how breaking news happens, because her description of her typical workday offered a glimpse into her news agency's radio room. Radio rooms are the site in newsrooms in which reporters identify and track breaking news stories. According to Laura, they are also the setting where texts from police enter into reporters' newswork:

> So, in breaking news there's what's called the radio room. Originally there was a bunch of police radios and paramedic radios ... but they stopped working, I think it was about two years ago when the police decided that the media wasn't allowed to listen to these radios anymore and now it's not legal or something, I don't actually know, but they don't work anymore. So, we have all these radios that don't really work, so we can't really listen, you used to be able to hear every single call, so now we can't do that so now we really rely on police, their tweets and what they give out to us.

In this description, Laura historicizes her newswork and situates her work practices within the changing conditions of breaking news reporting. Since the early 2000s, police forces have switched to digital radios and encrypted their signals, citing the safety of police officers, public safety, and citizen privacy as reasons to block outside parties from listening in. Before police encrypted their signals, reporters might, for example, hear of a robbery in progress and then develop a news report of the robbery based on the communications they heard police having over the radio. As Laura's comments make clear, now that police radios have gone silent, her newswork depends on reading texts that police communications divisions distribute online. When Laura reads tweets and news releases from police, these texts instigate the reporter's newswork practices in particular ways:

> So, you're monitoring breaking news sources, so it's mostly monitoring breaking news from police so if there's something going on ... police will tweet it, they do a good job of updating their tweets and letting the public know what's going on and then we follow up with ... Police, sometimes paramedics, firefighters, sometimes there's witnesses who post things on social media, "I saw this fire," "I saw this car crash." We monitor social media for updates like that. You update an article that you write that's posted online, that's also what I do. Sometimes it's relating, rewriting press releases from police, trying to find people on social media that police haven't identified.

This quote illuminates that police texts shape how an event comes to be known to reporters as a crime story. For example, it is striking that

Laura's conception of "if there's something going on" is based on messages that police produce and circulate on Twitter. It is also noteworthy that in this description, the reporter seems to understand that police are responsible for an activity that is typically associated with journalism: "letting the public know what's going on." Reading this segment for how the speaker's work is socially organized involves attending to the forms of activity that are represented in her talk and to the relations that make that activity possible (Mykhalovskiy and McCoy 2002, 29). Thus, consider the range of newswork practices that occur as Laura activates a police tweet: Her reading of the police's account of a news event directs her to conduct follow-up interviews with first responders and to monitor social media for posts by individuals who witnessed the event that police reported. The police tweet also incites Laura to write. Laura describes that once a news release is published by police, she may rewrite it, post the article online, and then update the article as more information is made available.

The reporter's comments start to demonstrate how police texts act not only as a way of knowing about a news event, but almost as a standardized set of instructions for how to report an event as a crime story. The details included in the news releases provide the reporter with a textual foundation upon which she crafts a news story. The way that Laura understands the police texts through the language of instruction emerged when she stated, "now it's more like police tells you what the story is, like you don't really have that much of a decision anymore." Another reporter, named Diana, echoed this understanding of police news releases as a sort of instructive document. She confirmed that reporters

> definitely react to press releases, but I wouldn't feel like I was really doing my job properly if that was the only way I was developing stories, because that's only the stories that the [police] administration want you to know, and there's often other more interesting ones, or more nuanced ones.

Police texts announce to the public and the press that they have criminally charged an individual and provide reporters with the details of an event that they then assemble into a news story. It is not as though the reporter is out in the world independently gathering facts. Instead, the reporter's work centres on reading and writing practices that build news from the textual foundation of police documents. This suggests that police texts are instrumental to courses of action that produce standard crime genre stories about HIV criminalization.

My interview with Laura brought into view particular ways that policing knowledge is pulled into journalists' writing. She provided a detailed account of the steps that she took to produce a news article about a man who faced charges related to not disclosing his HIV-positive status to sex partners:

> I got an email from police, it was a press release. I get emails for every press release they send out. I read it, HIV non-disclosure incident in downtown core. Usually if it's in the downtown core, we usually write about things that happen in the downtown core, I forwarded it to my editor and said "do you want to write about this? We wrote about this person back in 2014 or 2015 when the first charges were brought forward."
>
> My editor got back to me and said, "yes do a follow up." It's always responsible for us to do a follow up on stories to keep updated. After that I wanted to get more information from police, so I called them … whoever was on shift at police wasn't answering me, sometimes they're really busy. It wasn't like I really needed to talk to anyone because they issued a press release, I called them a few times and they didn't get back to me, so I just wrote it up. Pretty much re-worded the press release to make it coherent, straightforward … yeah, you upload the photo that … also goes in the press release, and then we just send it off to the online editors and the editor, the senior editor, whoever is on during that shift, for them to read it over, and then it goes online, that's pretty much it.

This quote offers a glimpse into the everyday work activities of a breaking news reporter and makes visible three ways that the speaker's newswork is coordinated with policing work. First, the police's account of the event makes it possible for the reporter to produce a news article that is structured as a standard crime story. The article that Laura wrote includes a mug-shot style photo of the accused and relies heavily on details included in the police news release, including the approximate geographic area in which police allege the crime was committed, the approximate date at which police allege it took place, and details regarding the next steps in the criminal-legal processing of this case.

Laura's earlier remarks, about how she understands that the police tell her what the story is, resonate in this passage. The reporter is made aware of this case through a police news release and the content and form of the police text shapes her understanding of the event as a type of crime. Other journalists who I interviewed helped me to appreciate how police press releases can filter a reporter's perspective on an issue.

For example, one experienced journalist described that when she first started working in a newsroom as an intern years ago, her

> job was to create a constant flow of copy for the website … like just little cop reads. Those were heavily reliant on press releases from the cops … they're two hundred words long, not a lot of room for nuance or context at all … HIV non-disclosure was always covered as a crime if the police think it's a crime … the cops say this is a crime, and you say oh god this is a crime, crime is bad, this person is a bad person.

In this passage, and in Laura's account above, the police texts that enter into reporters' work routines provide the raw material for journalists to write about "HIV non-disclosure incidents" as a type of crime story about a "bad person." The police texts include the name and image of a person facing a criminal charge, a specific location at which the alleged criminal activities occurred, and other details that a reporter can efficiently transfer into news content in the form of a "little cop read." Thus, police news releases operate, on one level, as an important source of information for reporters.

A second important aspect of Laura's account of her newswork is that it begins to show that police texts also enter into reporters' newswork practices in a much more complex way than acting simply as sources of information. Rather, Laura's description of her work with the police text provides a way to understand police news releases as coordinators of inter-professional relations in which journalists incorporate the police's understanding of public safety and crime into their newswork. Laura's newswork, in the passage above, centres on writing activities that recontextualize the police text as a news article. The police published the news release as part of an effort to build a case against the individual they had charged; however, Laura repurposes the document by extracting aspects of the text and fitting them into her newswork routines. As she imports the police news release into her professional setting, she strategically selects and endorses parts of the police text that fit journalists' professional perspective. For example, she related the police text to news articles that her news organization has published about this individual in the past and connected segments of the police text to journalistic standards of the "public interest."[2] Laura described

---

2 Laura drew on particular guidelines listed on her news organization's website as a text-based source of her understanding of what it means for a news story's publication to be in the "public interest." I have not included the text here so as to protect the anonymity of the participant and her news organization.

that the police text met standard journalistic criteria of public interest because:

> the location [in which the criminal charge was laid] is of public interest because the incidences happened with a number of women in the down-town core, there were multiple victims, so that is a consideration that should be written about in the public interest, we had written about the case before, so making sure the story is up to date, and it's a sexual assault, it wasn't consensual, so it's something that should be written about.

Her work activities to recontextualize the police document as a news story exemplify how the discourse of particular categories of professionals blend together when communicative content is handled across professions (Linell 1998, 150).

The third significant feature of the reporter's account of her work with the police text has to do with how the document coordinates newswork and police communications work in a particular way. Police news releases typically direct readers to contact an individual in the corporate communications division of the police force to access more information about the case. This aspect of the document is noteworthy, because it is another way that reporters' newswork reproduces the institutional relations of police communications work. Shawn, a reporter who regularly works with police news releases, explained how contacting police officers listed on police press releases for information often disrupts the specificity of his journalistic voice:

> Most of the media will just go straight to the spokesperson, but that makes me a little uneasy because ... basically the spokesperson gets to do my job for me where they ask the questions they think are relevant to the lead investigator, they compress them into a set of talking points that I'm sure have been vetted up and down. Their worry is that anything they tell me could, if charges are being laid, could compromise the investigation in some way. So they're very careful. This means you usually get this terse cop speak.

This account offers an interesting example of how police communications work enters into the realm of newswork. Shawn's practice of activating the contact information on the police document inserts him into the organizational structure of police in which a spokesperson supplants Shawn's reporting work. It is unsurprising that interviews that are filtered by a police spokesperson reproduce the restrictive "cop speak" of police news releases. Reporters I interviewed often described that police spokespeople are challenging to reach and that they are often left to rely on the text of news releases anyway. This was the case in Laura's article about the HIV non-disclosure case in which she described that "whoever was on shift at police wasn't answering me" and so she "pretty much re-worded the press release." In so doing, Laura's actions exemplify how reporters' activities discursively facilitate the relations of police, by making it possible for police texts to cross professional boundaries, coordinate crime reporting, and to appear in multiple local sites at which news articles circulate in print and online.

"Those Are Our Facts": The Coordination of Newswork and Police Work

To better understand how news reports of HIV criminalization happen, I wanted to know more about how the police texts that reporters depend on are produced and circulated. A thorough understanding of how news reports on HIV criminalization happen requires that one attend not only to the work that journalists do to process texts into news reports, but also the work of those who create the texts that journalists activate. Learning more about how the police produce and distribute texts to journalists proved to be a challenging and somewhat awkward experience.

The Institutional Ethnographer as "VISITOR"

Scrolling through the pictures on my phone recently, I happened upon a photo that I forgot I had taken of myself an hour or so before I interviewed David, a supervisor in the corporate communications division of Regional Police Services (RPS). As a general rule, I'm not one for taking selfie pictures. But, peering at my reflection in the mirror above the sink in the police station's washroom, I couldn't help but snap one of me wearing a very brightly coloured, and quite official looking, visitor's badge. The moment felt like it was worth commemorating. I probably didn't require a badge around my neck that read "VISITOR" in large block letters to signal to others at the police station that "I don't work here." It was not just that I was the only one who was wearing a backpack instead of a police uniform, it had more to do with how I felt as though I somehow "lost" in every interaction I had with an officer that day; officers who spoke louder than I did and seemed much more confident, assertive, and self-assured than I felt in that space. I did, however, take something close to pride in that visitor's badge, because it might as well have been a medal in recognition of ethnographic persistence. It took me several tries to arrange the interview with David. In the months leading to our meeting, I exchanged no fewer than eleven emails and four phone calls with various people who work in the corporate communications department at RPS. I was finally able to confirm an interview by evoking the language of institutional ethnographic interviews to express that I was simply looking to have a conversation with someone in the department about what they do every day and wanted to learn more about how police news releases are produced. Finally, a representative of the RPS corporate communications division arranged my interview with David, the director of the division, on the condition that I send RPS the list of the questions that I planned to ask during the interview, and "because you're not looking for perceptions or opinions, only facts." The conversation that I had with David brought into clearer view the extent to which the police understand themselves to be in the business of disseminating facts.

My social position as a white graduate student afforded me the privilege of navigating the police station and interacting with police officers on their home turf with ethnographic curiosity, with a sense of adventure, accompanied by moments of feeling intimidated and annoyed but not unsafe. It is likely that my whiteness, maleness, and class position make me a less startling type of "VISITOR" in this space of law enforcement. Around the time of my interview at the police station, I had attended a community event to mark the launch of Robyn Maynard's disquieting book *Policing Black Lives*. I wondered how the officers I walked by and spoke with at the station would respond to the types of questions posed to the panel of speakers during the question and answer portion of the book launch. Questions that were obviously more embodied and urgent than those I listed in the email I sent to RPS for approval. Questions along the lines of, "as a social support worker, I work with women who are being tortured, brutalized by police, called the 'N word,' called 'bitch,' what strategies do those of you on the panel have for assisting women in this position?" and, "If I'm stopped by police and carded, can I refuse to give my ID?" to which panellists responded that they advise those in the audience to "do what you have to do to survive the encounter."

After signing in at the front desk I was directed to a waiting area, and then to another waiting area, and then to a phone on the wall to speak to an officer behind plexiglass, who came and showed me to David's office. Once I finally made it into David's office, the steps towards the interview did not immediately become easier. David invited me to sit at a round table that was empty, save for the interview questions I had sent RPS placed neatly in front of his seat. I started by handing David my informed consent document as confidently as I could. I was used to this portion of interviews being rather brief and informal, but David very carefully and deliberately examined the document line by line. I then commenced the interview by promptly fumbling the first question: "so maybe you can start by telling me about what corporate services ...," David interrupted and impatiently corrected me, "corporate communications." "Right, sorry, corporate communications, what is involved in that department's work?"

Facts as Coordinators of Police Work and Newswork

My interview with David helped me to better understand the process through which news releases are produced and inserted into the work sequences of reporters. As he described, the catalyst for the production of a news release

> can come from a division, it can come from a homicide squad, the holdup squad, sex crimes, fraud, it can come from anywhere. So, it's either a phone call asking about a news release, or it can be a news release that comes to us, one of my media relations officers will look at what they've given us and put it in our template. We have templates for, there aren't that many types of news releases, so we've had for years, templates so that you don't have to reinvent the wheel every time. The media also knows exactly what they're getting. They know what information will be there, how it's laid out etcetera. [A police officer will] put together a news release and then in most cases it will come to me to be reviewed and authorized. I mean technology has changed, it's now, news releases are posted on our website and then automatically posted to our main Twitter account and to our main Facebook account.

In this passage, David explains that his department's production of a news release can be instigated either by a request from a particular division of the police force or by an officer who works in the corporate communications division. David's remarks suggest that constructing press releases involves selecting details that help police to do investigative work (such as identifying new complainants) and fitting them into standard templates[3] that the corporate communications division

---

3 I emailed David following our interview to request to see a blank template that the corporate communications division would use, but I was unable to obtain one. He responded: "I'm not able to provide you with a blank template. Can I suggest you look at the 30 days' worth of releases on our website and you will be able to see for yourself how releases are put together?"

uses to format their accounts. The final step is to circulate the news release on social media platforms. David's remarks imply that news releases are not simply intended to enlist the public in policing, they are produced in a form that anticipates and aligns with the information that reporters require to make news stories. To help me gain a better sense of what a standard news release template looks like, David placed a template that would be used in the event of a missing person on the table in front of me and described how police use the document. This exercise offered important insight into how a template structures the way that facts pertaining to a missing person case are organized into a news release:

> The point is that, and the argument that I use is that it saves time, you have consistency, but also for the media, use the example, if you go into Burger King, a Whopper will be the same thing here or anywhere else or a Holiday Inn, it's no surprises. So, a missing person says, the template says missing in brackets, man, woman, whatever, location, name, age, requesting assistance locating a missing, fill-in the whatever the person is, name, age, last seen, when they were last seen, where, map reference, description, sometimes there is a concern for safety for more reasons than others, anyone with information for more news and you fill it in. So, every missing man is going to look like that.

The document provides a standard text that is used to publicize the event of a missing person. While some segments of the document, such as "police ask for the public to assist with locating ..." are common to all press releases about missing persons, other segments are left blank so that officers can include specific information about the case, such as the missing person's name, age, sex, the location at which they were last seen, the time at which they were last seen, and a description of the person's appearance.

David's account of the template helped to make clear how the textual mechanics of the police news release operate to organize and standardize how the facts of a case are made available to reporters. In the segment above, David represents the news release as a standardized resource that facilitates journalists' access to pertinent information upon which they can craft a news text. He understands the standardized news releases as texts that make reporters' work more efficient:

> I mean they, it strikes me as common sense, and it was to them too, if I give you something in a standard form that makes it easier for you to do your job, you will respond positively. If you're getting a dog's breakfast of stuff,

I mean it's the basic human reaction, if I make your job easier to do, you will respond positively.

As David anticipated, many reporters I spoke with related to news releases as documents that make their work more efficient. Reporters consistently explained that they rely on police texts as a news source that they can efficiently transfer into widely spreadable news content at the rapid pace converged news organizations require. News releases also coordinate journalists' understanding of the facts of a case. Reporters described that they use police news releases as the foundational account of, to put it simply, what happened. For example, a breaking news reporter named Jessica (who works in the same radio room as Laura) explained that her work involves translating the facts that structure a news release into news articles: "we're reporting facts, so if the police put it in a very boring, robotic, you know this happened at this time, we have to go by that, those are our facts, we can't pull anything or assume anything." As the reporter's remarks imply, the facts that police distribute often become the facts that reporters circulate in news articles. Jessica's comments also start to show that reporters can struggle with the way news releases constrict and narrow their activities to report news. In this instance, the reporter finds that news releases constrain her writing and make it a more robotic, less interesting practice. For Jessica, there is less journalism writing and newswork to do in a context in which the facts that police distribute become "our facts."

Jessica seems to grapple with the tension between what has been referred to as the "objectivity norm" in journalism and her desire to convey her unique, journalistic voice in her news writing. As Marcel Broersma (2010, 28) explains, "the objectivity norm prescribes neutrality and only the transmission of facts … Reporters have to write in a detached tone … it has become a central concept in journalism's collective discourse." Jessica's remarks about "reporting facts" that police publish in a "boring, robotic" tone suggest that she is hesitant to muddy the facticity of her news account by "making a story" out of it. Her perspective echoes ethnographic studies of news production that focus on journalists who believe that "the facts should speak for themselves" and dislike the practices of "jazzing them [factual accounts of news] up" because it would violate the practice of truth telling (Boesman and Meijer 2018). For Jessica, transferring police talk into a news article is a way to achieve facticity and satisfy the objectivity norm.

Other reporters recounted similar experiences as Jessica to describe how the realms of police communications work and newswork can mesh in the process of producing a news story. Consider, for example, how a veteran reporter named Joan explained the delicate balance that she believes reporters must strike in their relationship with police:

> So, once you are embedded you are on their [the police's] side, you're suddenly telling the stories as they [the police] see them, as they want you to tell them … I think mostly you're not even aware that's happened, you still would feel like you're covering the story the way that you have always, but you wouldn't start to see that you were picking up the police perspective, the police viewpoint, from being too close to them. So, you really need to somehow be at arm's length from the police when you're covering police stories. You need to listen to them, be respectful, and then do all your own checks around, what does the victim say? What does the perpetrator say? What's the context of this? What does the court say? You need to chase down all the things because police are ultimately, I mean, sure, they can say there was a collision at this corner at this time of night. That's a fact, there was a collision at this corner at this time of night. Everything else? It really, quickly gets into conjecture and you can, you have to be really, really careful that the police opinion of that accident and words that they use to describe the people involved in it are not becoming part of your story.

In this passage, the reporter's remarks demonstrate another way that police communications work and newswork come together to produce factual accounts of an event. Whereas Jessica tries to maintain an objective stance and relies on police as the type of credible, authoritative source whose statements can be quoted to establish facts (Ericson 1988), Joan describes how she recontextualizes the police account of an event and turns it into a news story. Instead of opposing stories and facts, Joan considers storytelling as a tool to articulate the facts of a case more truthfully (Boesman and Meijer 2018, 1002). The speaker's remarks are interesting because they reveal that the information that police distribute to reporters not only provides a source of news stories, it also makes other actions within the realm of journalism possible. For example, the work that police do to distribute the factual information that "there was a collision at this corner at this time of night," makes it possible for journalists to do the work of investigating, identifying other sources, and providing contextual depth to news stories about the event.

Constructions of Public Safety as Coordinators of Police Work and Newswork

Up to this point, the coordination of police communications work and newswork may seem relatively uncomplicated. David, Jessica, and Joan describe a sequence of activities in which an event occurs, police distribute information about that event, and reporters take on the facts provided in the police's account, but may also add additional depth, context, and perspective to a news story. However, reading interview transcripts for social organization shows that reporters' work with police press releases not only recontextualizes the polices' factual account of an event as news, it also recontextualizes police knowledge and forms of reasoning that construct and attach meaning to people. Consider David's explanation of the criteria that his department follows for producing a news release:

> Well, there has to be a reason. Last year we probably did … a fraction of the people we arrest, we don't do them all, there has to be a reason, there has to be we're looking for someone, we have a description, we have a picture, this person has escaped custody and poses a threat to the community, this person is attacking women in their forties in this part of the city. There has to be some investigative value to it … if it's a threat to public safety it goes out right away, even if it's the middle of the night. Because we have an obligation, if there's a threat to public safety, to get that information out as quickly as we can.

In this passage, the speaker describes how press releases facilitate the work of policing and solicit the public's assistance in investigating crimes. David also understands the circulation of news releases as part of the police's broader mandate to protect public safety. David's remarks show that police news releases do more than simply organize facts about a crime into a standard template (this crime occurred at this time at this place); police news releases also work to produce the person named in the text as a public safety threat. This construction of a person as a public safety threat is accomplished in news releases by pairing one's name, photo, personal information, and descriptions of criminal charges they face with language that underscores the danger that one poses to others. For example, in the news release that pertains to the man facing charges related to allegedly not disclosing his HIV-positive status to sex partners, the text emphasizes that "police are concerned there may be more victims." This sort of language not only constructs the person facing charges as a threatening figure, it also acts as a signal to reporters who are sifting through various news releases throughout their workday that this particular item is newsworthy. For example, as Jessica described how she identifies a newsworthy story when working in the radio room, she explained:

> I think you develop a pretty good intuition for it through the years. But police will also put out press releases, for example, if they're looking for

someone involved in a crime, they'll say, they might say very clearly that there is a huge public safety element. They won't say it in those words, they won't spell it out, but it's pretty understood if you read between the lines. Or they'll say that the police are concerned that there may be more victims, police are warning people that this person is armed, do not approach. Language like that is a really good indicator for us.

In this passage, Jessica's assessment of newsworthiness is coordinated by the language that police employ to produce an individual as a public safety threat. Her work as a reporter is connected to the work of police as she takes up and circulates descriptions of individuals that police construct as threatening figures. The implications of this type of coordination of police communications work and newswork become weightier as one considers that police understand news releases as powerful policing instruments that can be used to surveil, monitor, and regulate those they deem threats to public safety. David recounted:

We started a thing a few years ago, and I'd love to tell you that we knew this was going to happen, but we now see regularly criminals surrendering shortly after we put their pictures up. And if you think about, if our main account we reach thousands of people, but if a news organization with 1.75 million retweets, it means everyone in the city is going to get it. And I would love to be there when someone sees their face come up on their phone. Our record in homicides is one hour, we had a man whose lawyer said don't do anything until police start looking for you. We put his picture out and three hours later he's at the front counter saying, "I'm your guy." That's amazing, I never thought that would happen, and that's the most satisfying, out of all the stuff that we do, that's the most satisfying because no one expects us to be able to get homicide investigation to surrender, and these things are very expensive and very time consuming.

David's vision of how police news releases latch on to the platforms that news organizations use to disseminate news suggests that police also employ online news as an instrument for more efficient policing. When reporters rely on police news releases and structure their newswork upon these texts, their activities are closely related to other forms of ruling that shape the experiences of those who are criminalized, including people who live with HIV and face charges related to not disclosing their HIV-positive status.

Consider Jessica's account of her newswork to produce a news story about a man facing criminal charges for not disclosing his HIV-positive status to sex partners:

So, this is written straight from a press release ... there are issues of stigma for using photos of people with HIV, but this guy has sexually assaulted (allegedly) a number of people, so I feel like public safety outweighs his personal privacy at this point ... there had been a lot of victims, so if people didn't know his name when they had relations with him, they might be helped by a photo.

The reporter's comments show how the criteria of public safety set out by police structure her news story about HIV criminalization. In this case, the name, photo, and HIV-positive status of this individual were disseminated in the mainstream press because the reporter wrote the story "straight from a press release." Furthermore, her understanding of the case's newsworthiness is coordinated by policing concepts such as "public safety" and motivated in part by an effort to enhance the public surveillance of this individual in order to encourage people to come forward and lay additional criminal charges. In the previous section, Jessica remarked that she understands her work as a reporter to consist of "reporting facts" that police distribute. When she described that the police's facts are "our facts," she evoked "our" as a first-person possessive pronoun to explain how she and her colleagues take up and use the facts that police distribute. However, it is important to keep in mind that when reporters circulate the police's construction of individuals as public safety threats "straight from a press release," those constructions become "ours" in a much broader sense as well. Large segments of the population do not have first-hand experiences of the criminal legal system, HIV disclosure, or the science of HIV transmission. Thus, their understanding of the connection between HIV, crime, public safety, and risk is heavily informed by mediated information (Henry and Tator 2002; Khan 2014; Mykhalovskiy et al. 2021b). The concern, of course, is that news reports based heavily on police texts instruct readers to relate to people living with HIV as threatening, security risks in need of regulation and control.

The Mainstream Press and the Expansion of the Police Mission Creep

Scholars who explore processes of crime reporting and police communications often promote ways of thinking about the relationship between the press and the police as two opposing sides locked in a sort of power struggle. For instance, there is a collection of scholarship that argues that the police dominate interaction with news media and fundamentally define how the media act (Chermak 1995; Grabosky and Wilson

1989). From this perspective, the police exercise their authority to control what is presented in the news, and the press serve as conduits for police ideology. Researchers attribute the asymmetrical character of the relationship between the press and the police largely to the influence of police spokespeople who act as gatekeepers, controlling the information that journalists require to do their work (Chermak and Weiss 2005; Surette and Richard 1995).

Meanwhile, there is also a corpus of research that foregrounds ways that media determine the conduct of police (Chermak 1995, 24; Ericson, Baranek, and Chan 1989). For example, recent scholarship points out that online social media has exposed police misconduct in ways that can spark social movements that compel police forces to alter their practices (Brown 2016; Nix and Pickett 2017). This, of course, is clearly evident in the ways that the murders of George Floyd, Michael Brown, Eric Garner, and too many others at the hands of police being captured on social media amplified the Black Lives Matter movement and sparked extensive discussions about police funding and the broader role of policing in society.

Researchers also show that the press shapes how police communicate with the public. For example, studies demonstrate that police sources typically communicate information in a way that is consistent with media formats, logic, and editing (Chermak 1995, 24). This trend resonates with David's understanding of police news releases as templated documents designed to enter into reporters' work routines in a way that makes their newswork more efficient. Researchers suggest that police are willing to bend to meet the demands of the press, because police acknowledge that news media are an important site in which to do "legitimation" work (Chermak and Weiss 2005, 503; Ericson, Baranek, and Chan 1989).

Certainly, one could relate to the interview data included in this chapter as evidence of a sort of power struggle between the press and police. For example, there were instances in which reporters were bothered by ways that police usurped the work of determining what events count as newsworthy and selecting the facts that are made available to the public. At the same time, David expressed frustration with reporters who rejected the standardized way that police forces organize an account of a newsworthy event. However, my concern with conceptualizing the relationship between police and the press as a stark binary, or as a sort of power struggle, is that such an understanding writes over the ways that the activities of police and reporters are coordinated to circulate messages that construct certain individuals as public safety threats. Thus, in this chapter, my intent has been to encourage a more relational approach that shows how the coordination of police communications work and newswork is hooked into broader relations of ruling that shape the experiences of people who are constructed as threats to public safety.

An understanding of how various institutions come to be geared into relations of policing through their reliance on information that police produce and distribute is brought into clearer view through Richard Ericson's (1994, 151) conception of the police as "knowledge brokers." Ericson's study of policing practices identifies that officers actually spend relatively little time directly protecting people and property against criminal threats. He argues that it is most accurate to conceptualize police as "knowledge brokers, expert advisors and security managers to other institutions. It is knowledge for security that constitutes their trade. The police officer produces and distributes knowledge for the risk management activities of security operatives in other institutions." Conceptualizing the police merely as "knowledge brokers" risks overwriting the myriad ways that police enact violence, especially upon communities of Indigenous people, Black people, people of colour, women, migrants, trans communities, people without access to housing, people who use drugs, and people who sell sex. Nevertheless, recognizing that the production and circulation of risk knowledge across institutional boundaries is a primary police activity points to a significant way that police maintain and expand their influence.

For example, Ericson (1994, 152) describes how an officer's work to respond to an automobile accident consists mostly of activities to fill out forms that distribute knowledge to various institutions such as criminal courts, insurance adjusters, medical professionals, the motor vehicle registry, and persons involved in profiling risk in a way that can be used in accident prevention, traffic management, resource allocation, and automobile industry compliance. Ericson's understanding of police as knowledge brokers in this example directs attention to how information that police circulate instigates work activities to manage risk across a range of institutional settings.

Ericson argues that the police's role as knowledge brokers to other institutions is a central part of the contemporary "risk society" (Beck 1992; Giddens 1990, 1991). He understands the "risk society" to be one "characterized by institutions organized in relation to fear, risk assessment and the provision of security. These institutions – for example, insurance companies, social security agencies and regulatory agencies – refigure the community into communications about risk in every conceivable aspect of life" (Ericson 1994, 163). As the range of institutions that depend on the information that police distribute expands in a risk society, police activity ceases to correspond to a particular territorial setting, and police are able to move through myriad settings as security experts (160). This sort of expansion of police functions into new settings is commonly referred to as the police "mission creep" or "mission drift" (Wood 2014). For example, observers have expressed concerns about how police now address "security concerns" in expansive settings such as schools (Beger 2002; Monahan and Torres 2010; Theriot 2009), public transportation systems (Côté-Lussier 2013), mental health care, public housing, and public parks (Camp, Jordan, and Heatherton 2016).

I want to situate the mainstream press as a site that propels the police mission creep. This chapter shows that the conditions of digital news production position reporters to rely on police communication materials and transpose significant sections of police texts as news texts. For example, the accounts of reporters I spoke with illuminate that reporters (or news editors) will produce a headline for the article, add a caption to the police's mugshot, and assemble the bullet-point details from the police text into a narrative about what police have said and done. As an institutional ethnography, this study relates to such text-mediated work activities as practices that coordinate what people are doing in newsrooms with the work that police are doing in public relations departments. In the context of news about HIV criminalization, reporters' reliance on readily available digital police texts is likely to produce messages that equate HIV serostatus with notions of dangerous criminality, and as a long line of critical discourse analyses confirm, these messages often reproduce harmful gendered and racialized tropes.

More broadly, reporters' work with police communication texts makes the press an avenue for police to distribute information to a wide audience of news readers. Ericson's conception of the police as knowledge brokers describes a context in which the police mandate expands as police serve as expert advisors who provide information for risk management to an increasing range of institutions. However, the newswork practices made visible in this chapter amplify the ruling relations of police, because news mediums make it possible for the police's constructions of public safety threats to appear in multiple local sites at a given time. In this context, the police do not simply act as knowledge brokers, expert advisors, and security mangers to the sort of professional settings that Ericson describes (such as insurance companies, social security agencies, and regulatory agencies); instead, news media deliver police messages about risk and security to the everyday worlds of those who read, click on, scroll through, share, and tweet news stories. This means that information that police circulate not only coordinates how those who work in a range of settings respond to risk, police texts also shape how news audiences access, interpret, and respond to constructions of public safety threats in their everyday lives.

Thinking Relationally about Intersections
Between News Media and Police

As mentioned in chapter 1, institutional ethnographies often focus on the social organization of a particular institution. However, the accounts in this chapter clarify the need to trace how social relations are also coordinated across institutions such as news media and police. Because this sort of analysis is sometimes outside the scope of institutional ethnographic research, in this section of the chapter I offer some provisional thoughts on how institutional ethnographers might expand analyses to conceptualize intersecting ruling relations.

One way that institutional ethnographers might enhance analyses of ruling relations that cut across institutions is to place their work into conversation with studies of the medico-legal borderland, as well as works from the broader field of relational sociology. Stefan Timmermans and Jonathan Gabe, for instance, extend relational thinking by evoking the metaphor of a borderland to call attention to connections between medicine, health, and law. Borderlands are often experienced as a barrier or site of exclusion. Instead, Timmermans and Gabe (2002, 507) conceptualize the borderland as a space of intersection that requires tolerance for ambiguity and the challenging of established dualisms. The medico-legal borderland in particular highlights how contemporary jurisprudence and health care intersect at a densely populated, and often overlooked, borderland (507). As the authors describe:

> The borderland between crime and health care is populated and guarded by a number of professionals engaging in processes that contain both the criminalisation of contested medical interventions and the medicalisation of criminal danger. The medico-legal borderland has clinics, prisons, medical boards, courts, occupational and public health offices, regulatory government agencies, crisis intervention centres and street policing. The conjunction of legal and medical concerns thus occurs in specialised settings, such as the morgue of the forensic pathologist, where every action is defined in terms of a hybrid of legal and medical principles, or in places typically associated either with medicine or law enforcement such as jails or hospitals. What is typical of all these sites is that alliances are created that link medical knowledge with knowledge about criminal deviance for the purpose of social control. (507)

What is interesting about this passage is the way that it diverges from standard institutional ethnographic understandings of social relations. Timmermans and Gabe's discussion is not restricted to the formal elements of a given functional complex such as health care. Rather, their perspective extends to multiple institutional sites. This passage describes the medico-legal borderland as a space in which aspects of crime and health intersect but cannot be simply reduced as straightforward binaries (McClelland 2013). Here, we can start to see how conceptualizing social relations as a process in which features of disparate institutions intersect and adjoin as hybrids can support institutional ethnographers' thinking about how different institutions connect with one another. We know that IE can help enlarge the scope of people's understanding about how their everyday activities hook into the work that others do elsewhere. However, theorizations of the medico-legal borderland push institutional ethnographers to conceptualize social relations not only as a way to look at how an individual's work in one setting is connected to the work of an individual in another setting, but as social relations that cut across institutions and form entirely new hybrid identities, environments, and forms of ruling. For the present study, this means thinking about the relationship between the press and police not only in terms of how the activities of reporters in newsrooms are sequenced with the work of police communication officers in police stations, but to also consider how the institutions of news media and police mutually construct one another.

The work of relational sociologists is helpful for locating language to describe what it means to conceptualize news media and police as knotted together in this way. When reading this literature, one will find that relational sociologists regularly emphasize that relational sociology is not a unified theory or approach; however, they tend to agree that "the main point is that relational sociology reminds us that when we talk about 'societies,' 'social structures,' 'cultures,' or 'social things' … whatever we study and however we do it, the mode of production of social phenomena is based on relations between interactants" (Dépelteau 2018, 3; Emirbayer 1997, 285).

Relational sociologists might refer to the connection between the mainstream press and police communications as an "assemblage" in the Deleuzian sense. French philosopher Gilles Deleuze defines an assemblage as:

a multiplicity which is made up of many heterogeneous terms and which establishes liaisons, relations between them across ages, sexes and reigns – different natures. Thus, the assemblage's only unity is that of co-functioning:

it is a symbiosis, a 'sympathy'. It is never filiations which are important but alliances, alloys; these are not successions, lines of descent, but contagions, epidemics, the wind. (Deleuze and Parnet 1977, 69)

The notion of an assemblage has recently gained traction in journalism scholarship that conceptualizes the structure of news gathering as a sociotechnical assemblage (Ananny and Finn 2020). They argue that the news content that "digital first" organizations produce is determined less by individual reporters' relationships to particular sources, and as van Dijck and colleagues (2018, 58) write, "more by the interaction between the assemblage of news organizations, data services, and advertising networks that populate the contemporary news landscape." Ananny and Finn emphasize that assemblages of human and nonhuman actors – including data from other organizations – shape how online news is defined, produced, and circulated. The notion of online news as an assemblage is useful for directing analytic attention to the tremendous array of actors and technologies that collide to create the conditions under which digital news content is produced.

The notion of an assemblage is helpful for calling attention to how the blending of news media and police communications' practices, routines, and technologies form a distinct alloy. Recognizing the fusion of news media and police communications as a type of hybrid entity helps to get at the distinct, systematic means by which public knowledge about HIV criminalization is produced and circulated in the contemporary moment. This level of understanding can be lost when social relations are more narrowly understood as the sequenced work of an individual reporter and an individual police communications officer. In this sense, assemblages are also productive in that "they produce new territorial organizations, new behaviours, new expressions, new actors, and new realities" (Müller 2015, 29). Recognizing a news media/police assemblage directs the critical sociologist's vision to a range of new actors, new forms of ruling, and new consequences attached to digital data technologies that shape the contemporary context of HIV criminalization in Canada.

While scholarship on the medico-legal borderland can be helpful for directing the attention of institutional ethnographers to ways that different institutions intersect with one another, placing IE into conversations with such scholarship can also help to reduce the somewhat insular character of IE. One way that practitioners of IE often define the methodology is by distinguishing it from more mainstream or established approaches to sociology. Characterizing IE as an "alternative sociology" can be a productive way to underline the significance of developing inquiry from people's actual, everyday experiences instead of theoretical concepts and categories and advancing a materialist ontology of the social. At the same time, emphasizing the uniqueness and particularities of IE research can produce IE as an almost inward-looking and self-sufficient sociology that is wary of other approaches to sociological inquiry (Mykhalovskiy et al. 2021a). My hope is that by placing IE into conversation with other fields of sociology, this chapter demonstrates the analytic potential of flexible and adaptive IE research.

Responding to Intersections between News Media and Police

Throughout this chapter I've sought to bring into view the social relations that propel police knowledge and conceptions of risk and safety in the mainstream press. When considering the consequences of the police mission creep in the mainstream press, it is crucial to underline that state actors, such as police, protect some at the expense of others and work to maintain inequitable social, racial, and economic divisions (Maynard 2017). Within studies of public health, there is growing recognition among critical scholars that policing is antithetical to the social justice and emancipatory traditions of public health and the field's commitment "to fostering knowledge and shared power to promote health equity" (Fleming et al. 2021, 553). Critical researchers increasingly frame policing and law enforcement as an urgent public health issue (Alang et al. 2017; Boyd 2018; Cooper and Fullilove 2020; Garcia and Sharif 2015; Gilbert and Ray 2016; Krieger et al. 2015; Lopez 2019; Sewell and Jefferson 2016). As Fleming and colleagues (2021, 553) write, "policing practices have profound implications for death and illness, including direct and indirect physical and mental harm and violent practices that disproportionately target and harm Black, Indigenous, and Latinx residents." Many other groups, including Indigenous peoples, migrants, those who experience houselessness, the LGBTQ2S+ community, and those who experience mental distress, also experience heightened risk of police violence (554). Given this mounting evidence major public health and medical organizations (including the American Public Health Association and the American Medical Association) have recognized policing practices as a public health issue contributing to health inequities and in need of public health solutions (Spolum et al. 2023).

Accounts of newswork in this chapter reveal that talk and texts from police often circulate in mainstream news about HIV criminal non-disclosure cases in the name of "public safety." As the argument goes, widely circulating information about a person who police construct as a threatening public health risk can both deputize the public to support the police's efforts to build a criminal case against the individual and alert the public to the presence of a "risky" and "reckless" public health threat in their midst. However, critical public health scholarship that articulates policing as a longstanding threat to public health in and of itself, especially to communities made vulnerable by structural conditions, raises concerns about how sensationalist news reporting rooted in police discourse is likely to amplify harmful messages about HIV rather than effectively promote public health and safety. This means that as activists and researchers, we're confronted with the question of how to uncouple the press from police influence and how to preserve space for autonomous journalists who can hold police to account and speak truth to power.

As we envision paths to disentangling police and the press, we might consider two types of interventions. One approach might be best described as a discursive strategy that aims to re-frame crime genre stories as other types of news stories. Oftentimes this means advocating for an issue to be re-framed as less of a criminal law issue and more of a public health matter. Researchers who analyse media discourse around drug use, for example, have problematized the way that the issue is most often portrayed in the press as a criminal legal issue. Echoing many of the trends in news coverage of HIV criminalization, studies of media coverage about drug use consistently find that reportage emphasizes notions of punishment and prohibition, represents people who use drugs as threatening "criminal outsiders," and relies on alarmist imagery that accentuates risk, fear, and crisis (McGinty et al. 2016; Webster, Rice, and Sud 2020).

It is imperative to resist instances in which public health issues are framed as a kind of criminal identity. In addition to their highly damaging and stigmatizing quality, studies show that representations of "drug scares" and "moral panics" over-simplify the situation, individualize the issue, and reinforce and legitimize the use of coercive measures of control (Hughes, Lancaster, and Spicer 2011; Taylor 2008). As Webster and colleagues (2020) write in the context of the opioid poisoning epidemic, such emphasis on the activities of individual physicians or individual patients "leave us only with individual-level solutions" rather than broader public health responses (7). Considering these trends in news coverage, some scholars have called on the mainstream press to re-frame news discourse about opioids as public health stories. For example, Emma McGinty and colleagues' (2016, 405) study of news framing around opioids concludes: "Findings underscore the need for concerted effort to reframe opioid [use] as a treatable condition addressable via well-established public and behavioral health approaches."

In light of calls for crime stories to be re-framed as public health stories, it is worth pausing to consider the possible implications of such a discursive shift in the context of HIV criminalization. As described in the introductory chapter, recent directives from the Canadian government mean that criminal prosecutions for HIV criminal non-disclosure will likely continue to decline and that HIV disclosure will increasingly be governed by public health authorities. Fewer criminal charges related to HIV non-disclosure means that there will be fewer crime genre stories published and that when this topic does make its way into the press, news articles will likely often report on the activities of public health authorities.

There are important reasons to temper expectations that crime stories re-framed as public health stories will somehow be less stigmatizing or will diminish the forms of discrimination or "Othering" that pattern crime stories. People living with HIV have been hugely stigmatized and treated as villainous threats to public health within health news stories for decades. Contemporary health stories about HIV are likely to be a different register for producing stories that stigmatize people living with HIV.

Critical race scholars also remind us that establishing problematic connections between one's personal health and one's race or ethnicity is a very old pattern in Western societies (Reitmanova 2009, 185). Even if news reporting on HIV criminalization (or other issues) is re-framed as a public health news story, there is an ample body of literature that suggests that these news stories will remain catalysts for messages that produce racialized people and migrants as "Others" who pose a threat "to the highly regarded and healthy bodies of white Canadians" (Monson 2017, 4; Murdocca 2003, 24; Reitmanova 2009, 24). Negative health discourses about migrants and racialized communities consistently structure news coverage of public health crises such as the Ebola virus, SARS, and COVID-19 (Eichaelberger 2007; Gover, Harper, and Langton 2020; Greenberg 2000; Hier and Greenberg 2002; Murdocca 2003). This body of critical race scholarship is important because it prompts us to keep in mind that news reporting on public health issues reproduces many of the same troubling racist and stigmatizing patterns of crime reporting. With this in mind, sociological studies of public health news ought to centre race in their analyses and remain alert to ways that news reporting legitimizes the use of surveillance, regulation, and coercive regulation against BIPOC communities.

Given the limits of discursively re-framing crime genre stories, we might also consider more structural approaches to resisting stigmatizing news stories about HIV criminalization, such as expanding upon growing calls to #DefundThePolice. A focal point of calls to defund the police have justifiably been on the demilitarization of police forces. As organized movements contest the tools of physical police violence, it is important that the tools of symbolic police violence do not go unchallenged. Police communication infrastructures represent an important site of critique and divestment. Recently, calls to "defund the crime beat" have grown louder. As Tauhid Chappell and Mike Rispoli (2020) write, "while crime coverage fails to serve the public, it does serve three powerful constituencies: white supremacy, law enforcement, and newsrooms – specifically a newsrooms's bottom line." This book adds to a lineage of research that highlights the negative consequences of crime coverage (Beale 2006; Chappell and Rispoli 2020; Dixon 2018; Gramlick 2016).

The accounts in this IE study illustrate how reporters' reliance on police texts profoundly shape mainstream narratives of who poses a threat to public health and safety, and in the case of HIV criminalization in particular, instruct readers to relate to people living with HIV as safety risks in need of regulation and control. This type of discourse amplifies HIV stigma and helps to propel the criminalization of HIV that has shown to be out of step with public health and human rights principles. To this point, HIV activists have employed a range of strategies for dethatching police narratives from public discourse about HIV. This is an ongoing, urgent priority given that information that is published about an individual online exists as a digital object for indefinite periods of time. For example, in the jurisdiction in which David works, digital police press releases remain catalogued and publicly available on the police forces' website after one has served a sentence and even if the criminal charges are subsequently dropped. As David explained:

> our position is if what we said was accurate at the time it was published it stays there, if the charges were subsequently dropped, I mean that's a matter for the courts and the attorney general's ministry, we don't have the resources or anything to be able to maintain that. But if it was accurate at the time we published that you were charged with these offences then we won't take it down.

News stories that are based upon police news releases are typically published at the beginning of a criminal HIV non-disclosure case. In some instances, more news stories are published once a case proceeds to trial and news coverage about a criminal HIV non-disclosure case extends over weeks and months. These situations offer activists an opportunity to intervene in news coverage and to attempt to alter media messages about HIV and the criminal law. In the next chapter, activists describe the diverse approaches that they use to interrupt the coordination of police communications work and newswork.

Chapter Four

Activist Interventions

Thus far, my pursuit of understanding how the stable, standard genre of crime story about HIV criminalization endures has taken me to two empirical sites. In chapter 2, I introduced readers to the people who make news. Accounts from beat reporters, news editors, and freelance journalists illustrated ways that news production in an era of converged journalism is coordinated by relations of commercialization and generalist reporting. Reporters described the frenzied pace of their work within converged news agencies and the constant pressure that they face to produce news content that will attract a large online audience. In such a work environment, it is perhaps unsurprising that reporters recounted that in some cases, news production work is based largely on copy and pasting digital source texts into news articles. In chapter 2, I argued that these social conditions of contemporary news production contribute to the production of sensational accounts of topics such as HIV criminalization.

Chapter 3 furthered my analysis of the relations of news production by showing that a main reason that crime genre stories are a deeply engrained way of reporting on HIV non-disclosure is because reporters' work is closely coordinated with the work of police communications divisions. My interviews with journalists and someone who works in a police corporate communications division revealed that reporters' use of police press releases accelerates the flow of the police's definitions of crime, danger, risk, and security into public discourse. Because the publication of police press releases harms people who live with HIV who face charges, LGBTQ2+ groups, racialized communities, and communities of people affected by HIV, it is imperative for HIV advocates to prioritize the effort to separate police messages from public discourse about HIV.

In this chapter, I introduce readers to HIV advocates who take on the seismic task of intervening in mainstream news discourse and interrupting crime genre reporting about criminal HIV non-disclosure cases. The HIV advocates I interviewed do this work from different locations – as organizers of activist collectives, as lawyers working for non-governmental organizations (NGOs), and as executive directors of AIDS service organizations (ASOs). However, they share a common endeavour to shift the way that HIV criminalization, and people living with HIV, are represented in mainstream news. In place of the standard crime story genre that objectifies people living with HIV; portrays HIV non-disclosure as a straightforward, uncomplicated type of criminal offence; and sets readers up to view people who face criminal charges only as blame-worthy criminals, these advocates work to cultivate well-informed news stories that prominently feature their concerns about HIV criminalization and build momentum towards ending HIV criminalization.

This institutional ethnographic study of how HIV advocates intervene in mainstream news discourse is arranged into two parts. First, I present a news article in which advocates effectively interrupt standard crime genre reporting of a criminal HIV non-disclosure case. This news text illustrates the types of knowledge and critique that HIV advocates can insert into mainstream news discourse about HIV criminalization. Participants' descriptions of their difficult encounters with the mainstream press in this first section also help readers to appreciate what a tremendous feat it is to disrupt the standard way that mainstream news outlets have consistently reported on this issue for decades.

In the second part of this chapter, I draw on interviews with advocates who are active in efforts to change how HIV non-disclosure is covered in the mainstream press to argue that news coverage is not univocal. Social movements are a significant source of counter discourse and shape public knowledge by inserting their messages and critiques of HIV criminalization into news texts. In this chapter, I look closely at three types of work activities that participants described as they recounted efforts to shift media discourse on HIV non-disclosure: work as spokespeople, work to produce texts, and work to cultivate relationships with reporters.

Conversations that I had with fourteen HIV advocates who engage with news media in different ways, and from different locations, helped me to recognize that advocates' interactions with the press are highly complex accomplishments in social organization. Occasions when an HIV advocate interacts with a reporter as a spokesperson, or publishes an opinion editorial article, or points a reporter towards a newsworthy story, might seem like a simple interaction between a representative of an HIV organization and a news agency. However, I argue that participants' descriptions of their work in this chapter show that during their interactions with the press, advocates are actually coordinating diverse types of knowledge and expertise and aligning them with the relevancies of reporters' newswork. Advocates facilitate the production of news stories that feature their critiques of HIV criminalization by strategically providing reporters with material that they require to produce news stories, in formats that fit reporters' fast-paced news production routines. For example, accounts in this chapter show that advocates speak in interviews in ways that make their message easily quotable, produce texts that can be efficiently transferred into news texts, and support reporters' news selection activities by calling their attention to newsworthy events.

Intervening in Crime Story Reports of HIV Criminalization

As this book has shown, news reports about HIV criminalization have been written as straightforward crime genre stories for decades. Those who I spoke with for this chapter described the remarkable challenges they've faced while trying to disrupt such a stable and consistent genre of reporting. For example, John has been working with HIV activist groups for over twenty years. He recounted the condemning tone of news articles that were published at the time that one organization, The Ontario Working Group on Criminal Law and HIV Exposure (CLHE), was formed in 2007:

> Early on we were aware of media coverage that was problematic, focusing on specific cases and demonizing people and not getting at the issues that we were concerned about, particularly around, in the early years, around the science of transmission, around public health implications of using the criminal law, and so on. There was this moment, fairly early on, CLHE decided to have a public meeting; it was a meeting for people to discuss the issue, and it was meant for people living with HIV primarily, and their supporters ... There was over 100 people there and one of the things we didn't do is that we didn't determine in advance that it was closed to the media, nor did we ask people who were in attendance if they were representatives of the media. As it happened, Margaret Wente was in the audience, and she subsequently wrote a damaging, quite a long and damaging article about disclosure coming out of that meeting where she represented people living with HIV and the meeting at CLHE as a bunch of, you know, irresponsible people who want to spread HIV. So that was a real kind of wakeup call in terms of not having a lot of control over how the issue is represented and as a small organization,

volunteer organization we had very little power to intervene in how the media was framing the issue.

The speaker's comments make it possible to appreciate how crime genre stories can impede efforts to end HIV criminalization. As John points out, standard news reports are often sensational representations of HIV non-disclosure that demonize people living with HIV and erase the complexity of the issue. Not only is this type of news coverage highly stigmatizing, but it also writes over the serious concerns that activists have been expressing about HIV criminalization for years, such as how the law is out of step with current scientific research on HIV transmission and conflicts with public health and human rights principles.

The types of concerns that John raises are clearly evident in the news article by Margaret Wente (2008) that he refers to. For instance, Wente's article about CLHE's public meeting contends that the group engages in "the glorification of (highly risky) bareback sex"; "believes that everybody else should change except them"; and that "Toronto's AIDS establishment ... seem stuck in a swamp of victimology and denial." These aspects of the standard crime story genre that are present in Wente's article are noteworthy, because on this occasion, the author was not reporting on a particular criminal case. Therefore, the CLHE meeting was actually an opportunity for the author to write with a relative freedom from the constraints of the crime story genre and to produce a more nuanced and deeply researched news article. Nevertheless, the article features many of the well-worn, superficial, and sensational aspects of crime reporting about HIV non-disclosure. As John mentions, small volunteer organizations may feel as though they have little power to mobilize narratives that counter this sensational press coverage, because they lack the resources, media-relations expertise, or capacity to do so.

Unfortunately, at the time of writing, news reports about HIV criminalization are often structured by features of the standard crime story genre. For instance, troubling aspects of crime reporting were prevalent in coverage of two criminal HIV non-disclosure cases in November 2018. News reports of these cases circulated the content of police news releases, including photos and personal information of people living with HIV who face criminal charges related to non-disclosure. Reportage of these cases also reproduced stigmatizing and moralizing discourses in familiar ways. For example, they referred to people who live with HIV and face criminal charges related to HIV non-disclosures as morally culpable, "cruel and cavalier" (Richardson 2018). Nevertheless, it is important to acknowledge significant strides that HIV advocates

have made in their ongoing efforts to alter how the issue of HIV criminalization is represented in the mainstream press. For example, a long-
time activist named Steven described:

> What I find is that nowadays, unless it's one like the latest arrest, they
> [the news articles] usually have at least a line to say, "advocates have been
> protesting this," or something like that, so there is some sort of recogni-
> tion that there is a discussion about this, rather than "oh crazy person with
> HIV trying to infect people." And so that's a kind of improvement. Some
> of the articles are in that way relatively balanced, whereas at least you're
> there, where if you look back to the older stuff, in the first decade of the
> 2000s, there wasn't even an attempt [to include activists' perspectives in
> news articles].

Steven's comments start to make visible what an effective intervention
into the mainstream press might look like. For example, he recognizes
that contemporary articles feature activists' messages more often than
they did in the early 2000s. He also suggests that current reportage is
less likely to represent HIV non-disclosure as a straightforward offence
committed by objectified "crazy" people living with HIV. Articles that
diverge from the standard genre of crime story in this way are significant, because they equip news readers with information that they can
use to make sense of the issue of HIV non-disclosure – information that
is not regularly available to them in typical stories about HIV and the
criminal law.

For example, consider the ways that a news article from 2016, headlined "Advocates Hopeful Canada Will Stop Criminalizing Non-Disclosure
of HIV Status," written by journalist Joanna Smith, deviates from the
standard crime report about an HIV non-disclosure case. The article,
published in the Canadian Press, reports on a woman (who I will refer
to as M.S.) who was convicted of aggravated sexual assault in 2014
and was appealing her conviction in January of 2016. Between M.S.'s
arrest in 2013 and the eventual rejection of her appeal to have her sexual assault conviction overturned in 2017, there were nineteen news
articles published about this HIV non-disclosure case. Of these nineteen
articles, sixteen follow the standard pattern of criminal justice time: One
article is published when M.S. is initially charged (Turner 2013); when
she "lost her fight to get her case thrown out due to delay" (Turner 2014,
4); following the opening statements of her criminal trial (McIntyre
2014c); at the time of the trial's closing arguments (McIntyre 2014b);
and when she is found guilty (McIntyre 2014a). Ten news articles are
published throughout M.S.'s sentencing hearing. These news articles

rely exclusively on criminal legal system sources, including a police interview video played at trial; court rulings; and what the Crown, her defence lawyer, and witnesses called to testify (such as the defendant and a medical expert) say in court. Another news article is published when M.S.'s guilty verdict is upheld (May 2017).

In addition to criminal justice time reporting about M.S.'s case, the corpus of news stories also includes articles that centre advocates' voices and prominently feature their critiques of HIV criminalization. Two opinion editorial articles were published by legal experts who drew on documents and statements from the Canadian HIV/AIDS Legal Network[1] and the Canadian Coalition to Reform HIV Criminalization to problematize the use of the criminal law to respond to instances of non-disclosure. The other article that brings advocates' voices forward is the article by Joanna Smith (2016).

In some ways this news article written by Joanna Smith resembles the standard crime genre story about HIV criminalization. For example, the report situates the person facing criminal charges in a standard sequence of events through which criminal cases proceed. It also uses the language of the criminal justice system to write about her. The information about the person facing charges in the first part of the article is derived from a judge's ruling. Given that mainstream news has, for decades, consistently treated HIV non-disclosure cases (even the most complex cases) as straightforward crime stories, one might expect that the person facing charges would be portrayed as a morally blameworthy, reckless criminal in this news article. There are, however, meaningful ways that this piece deviates from the standard structure of news reports about HIV criminal cases. For example, the article includes important context that supports readers to acknowledge the complexity of HIV non-disclosure. In this instance, readers learn that the person facing charges was experiencing a difficult and volatile period in her life and that she feared that her HIV disclosure would lead to social isolation. By including these pertinent details, the reporter produces HIV disclosure as a complex, vulnerable, and arduous practice – a significant departure from typical crime reports that portray HIV non-disclosure simply as a reckless and decontextualized criminal act.

Another important feature of this news story is that critics of HIV criminalization have a strong presence throughout the article and express statements that shift the typical story line about HIV criminalization. It

---

1 Since I conducted this fieldwork, the Canadian HIV/AIDS Legal Network has changed the name of their organization to the HIV Legal Network.

is particularly significant that the perspective of advocates is expressed in the headline of the article, "Advocates Hopeful Canada Will Stop Criminalizing Non-Disclosure of HIV Status," because according to van Dijk (1988, 188–9), headlines function to define the most relevant information of the news item. He argues that because headlines "are often the only information read or memorized, they play an important role in the further information processing and possible effects of news."

The news article also includes quotations from former Justice Minister Jody Wilson-Raybould and legal experts that echo concerns about HIV criminalization that people living with HIV, HIV activists, and researchers have been expressing for years. These critiques have to do with how the laws used to prosecute HIV non-disclosure are out of step with current scientific evidence regarding HIV transmission, hinder public health efforts to address HIV, and enhance HIV stigma. For the purposes of the present study, it is especially noteworthy that the article includes a quotation that problematizes the way the news media typically report on HIV criminal cases, as lawyer Cynthia Fromstein states, "the only time you see HIV, practically, is when someone's picture is on the paper, being charged ... with aggravated sexual assault" (J. Smith 2016). The presence of this quote in the article signals an awareness of how news reportage of HIV criminalization exacerbates HIV stigma.

It would be difficult for those who read Joanna Smith's article in the morning paper, scrolled to it online, or shared it on social media to imagine the entire complex of activities that advocates carry out to help facilitate the production of this type of news text that prominently features their critiques of HIV criminalization. In the next section of this chapter, I look closely at how advocates produce and sustain a consistent critique of HIV criminalization in the press.

During my conversations with people involved in efforts to intervene in media representations of HIV criminalization, advocates regularly described the work they do when being interviewed by reporters, when producing texts that are intended to circulate in news media, and when fostering relationships with reporters. I related to advocates' descriptions of their work as windows into how their sustained presence in the press is made possible, the types of knowledge and expertise that need to be in place to produce media interventions, and how their work is positioned within broader organized responses to HIV criminalization.

Intervening in the Mainstream Press as Spokespeople

One of the primary ways that advocates' critiques of HIV criminalization gain traction in the mainstream press is through the work of those who take on the role of spokespeople and respond to reporters' requests to be news sources as interviewees. It is not surprising that advocates regularly described the practice of talking to reporters as a powerful way to shape news content about HIV criminalization. The news interview has been described as "the fundamental act" of contemporary journalism (Craig 2010, 75). For example, recall that in chapter 2 a harried daily news reporter named Alex explained that the very first step in his newswork process involved "looking for sources of people who are experts on the matter who can talk." Interviews in this section show that HIV advocates attract reporters' attention by producing themselves as certain types of experts who hold a specialized type of professional knowledge.

In this section, I draw primarily on interviews with advocates who work at the HIV Legal Network (LN). These conversations enabled me to explore how people working in an NGO insert their critiques of HIV criminalization into mainstream news discourse by connecting their professional knowledge and expertise to reporters' newswork practices. The work of the LN offers an example of one advocacy organization that has produced itself as a ready and reliable news source for reporters. Most of the reporters I spoke with understood the LN as an important voice to include in news reports about HIV criminalization. For example, reporters I interviewed described the LN in terms such as: the "usual characters," the "main organization," the "standard expert voice," and the "legal expertise that is really helpful" to contact when reporting on this topic.

The LN is not the only voice that is quoted in news reports about HIV criminalization. Over the course of this project, I spoke to representatives of activist groups, directors of ASOs, academic researchers, and people with lived experiences of HIV and/or criminalization who had been quoted in news stories. I focus on the work of the LN here, because my conversations with Richard Elliott, the organization's executive director, and Janet Butler-McPhee, the communications director,[2] were integral for my understanding of the particular way that spokespeople connect their knowledge and expertise to routine news production processes.

Before moving to my conversations with the executive director and the communications director, it is worth noting that the LN is a specific

2 In 2021, Richard Elliott stepped down as the executive director of the Legal Network after fourteen years. Janet Butler-McPhee and Sandra Ka Hon Chu were named co-executive directors.

type of NGO dedicated to promoting and protecting the legal rights of people living with HIV. At the time of my fieldwork, the organization employed twelve staff members, many of whom are lawyers who conduct policy research and analysis. The LN's main activities centre on efforts to repeal or reform laws and policies that discriminate against people living with HIV and other communities and populations particularly affected by HIV; to enact laws and policies that protect people living with HIV; and to support populations affected by HIV to understand and demand their human rights.

A unique feature of the LN that distinguishes it from other legal advocacy organizations, volunteer-led activist groups, and ASOs that also advocate to curb HIV criminalization is that it is equipped with resources and specialized expertise to respond to media interview requests. The following remarks from Richard, the executive director, help to bring into view what is required for HIV organizations to have a sustained presence in mainstream news:

> [The LN is] not just intervening in courts, but intervening in the court of public opinion, so engaging with media, trying to get media attention to the issue [of HIV criminalization] that we hope will be favourable. But also, responding to media inquiries that come in response to a particular prosecution going forward and becoming public knowledge. So then we also get called for some sort of reaction on the latest case ... If you look back twenty years ago, or even further to the beginning of the epidemic, the coverage was awful and that is less frequent now. And I think we've helped frame the terms of the discussion through some fairly relentless commentary in the media ... The concerns about criminal law are much more present now in the media coverage than they were ten or fifteen years ago.

Richard's comments start to suggest some of the ways that the LN has produced itself as a ready and reliable source of expert spokespeople on the topic of HIV criminalization. The organization is uniquely positioned to engage with the press, not only because they employ a communications director on staff, but also because they have had a sustained presence in the press for more than two decades. Over that time, they have developed strategies for interacting with the press in ways that amplify legal and human rights concerns about HIV criminalization. An important part of this strategy involves resisting the standard crime genre story that reporters are often prepared to write. As Richard describes:

> We ... get a call or the email out of the blue, saying, "hey, I want some comment on case x" that's about to be reported or has just been reported

[by police] ... or sometimes we already know that something's coming and
so we can anticipate that we'll get some media requests, like case x is going
to an appeal ... We generally try to avoid commenting on cases ... and try
to shift the focus of our remarks to the issue about why we have concerns
about over-criminalization and public health concerns, human rights concerns ... why we have these concerns about police doing this or why we
need to actually narrow the scope of the criminal law because a whole slew
of cases are caught up in the criminal justice system that shouldn't be.

The executive director's remarks display an acute understanding of
the intricacies of news media interviews. His comments acknowledge
that interactions with reporters are a complicated and distinct type of
communication event that differ from ordinary conversations. Communications scholar Geoffrey Craig (2010, 79) identifies that ordinary
conversation is defined by certain features, such as a sense of equal
status between participants, equal rights to speak, degrees of reciprocity, and assumptions about equal contributions to the conversation.
Meanwhile, news media interviews are a particular type of institutional
dialogue that is more goal oriented and involves obvious status dif-
ferences between participants with unequal access to information and
knowledge and unequal degrees of participation.

Richard's reflection on his experiences fielding calls from reporters
suggests that it is next to impossible to completely impede reporting
about HIV criminalization that is occasioned by criminal cases. There
is no way for HIV advocates to stop reporters from covering cases that
go to court, and therefore the bulk of reporting on this topic is inscribed
with criminal legal discourse. Perhaps the only way to fully interrupt
news stories that are patterned by the standard criminal justice processing of a case is to change the laws that are used to prosecute HIV
non-disclosure and stop cases from moving through the criminal justice
system in the first place.

What Richard's comments show is another way that advocates
attempt to limit the production of crime genre stories while they work
towards changing the criminal law itself. This strategy takes the form
of disrupting the institutional relevancies and language that structure crime genre stories and shifting the focus of the conversations
away from a particular individual and their case and towards broader
structural issues related to HIV criminalization. Richard's comments
above put into view the divergent goals of the reporter who requests
a comment on a criminal HIV non-disclosure case and the advocate-
spokesperson at the LN. While the reporter is seeking a comment about
a standard development in the criminal justice system's processing of

a case, Richard's goal is to resist contributing to a criminal justice narrative and to shift the conversation to advocates' concerns about HIV criminalization on the grounds of human rights and legal concerns. In order to shift reporters' attention to these critiques, advocates at the LN leverage their position as professionals who possess expert knowledge of policy analysis, advocacy, and litigation related to HIV and have access to the information that reporters require to craft news stories about HIV criminalization.

Janet, the LN's communications director described that she understands the work of being a spokesperson as akin to "a dance, the idea that at different points in the conversation, people will lead and follow, your challenge is to not have the journalists lead all the time." In order to help me better understand how she choreographs this dance with reporters, Janet walked me through how she responds to reporters who call the LN looking for comments about a criminal HIV non-disclosure case, and shifts the conversations to her organization's critiques of HIV criminalization:

> If I got a call like that, I never answer questions right away, I usually, I make an excuse, "I've got to be somewhere in ten minutes, tell me what you're asking about and I'm sure I can find someone to speak to you, but you have to give me ten minutes because I'm doing something else." I tend to take down the information and then, you know, my first reaction is to go to the researchers, and we come up with a plan. If it's a case like that, we would tend to, the good thing about legal cases is that you often have an out and you can say, "we don't know the case or the facts, so we can't speak to the facts of the case." So that gives you cover: "what I can tell you is some context, some more background on what you'll need to write about this." And usually they're quite happy with that, and usually that will help in terms of what the story ultimately looks like.

An important feature of her response is that it is largely an exercise in trying to introduce the analyses, research, and critiques that advocates at the LN have produced about HIV criminalization to a reporter, despite the fact that the reporter has not requested this information. If Janet's interaction with the reporter was a conventional conversation based on degrees of equal participation and reciprocity, she may feel inclined to respond to the particular questions the reporter asks. What is striking about the communications director's account is the way that she leverages the conventions of the news media interview and her position as an expert source with access to specialized knowledge and information.

In an effort to insert LN'S perspective into news reporting, Janet answers a reporter's phone call, makes an excuse to avoid responding to questions about a criminal case, gathers information, meets with researchers, plans how to reply to the reporter's questions, and responds to reporters by providing the relevant context she and others at LN believe should be included in news reports about HIV criminalization. What these activities accomplish is the coordination of research and analytic work at the LN with the reporter's need to include quotes from expert sources in news articles about HIV criminalization. As Janet describes, "saying just, 'no comment,' it makes it look worse than it is. Our goal in this is, even if we can't say exactly what they want us to say, is to say something that will help them. So that's my approach, my approach is I'm trying to help the media." The robust research and analytic work of the LN provide Janet with background information and context that make it possible for her to maintain the organization's status as a ready and reliable expert source on the issue of HIV criminalization, and at the same time centre longstanding human rights, public health, and social justice concerns about HIV criminalization.

Thus far we have seen how those at the LN leverage their status as expert spokespeople in an effort to interrupt crime genre reporting of HIV criminalization. My interviews suggest that another important way that the LN has established itself as a dependable source for reporters is by supporting people who have lived experiences of HIV and/or criminalization to draw on their expertise in order to take up the position of spokespeople in the press. Reporters, legal experts, and community-based activists who I interviewed often lamented that there are not more people with lived experiences of HIV and/or criminalization with an active presence in mainstream news discourse about HIV and the criminal law. The executive director of the LN explained:

> Media often ask for that too, "give me the human story, give me the individual who can speak this," and I get why they want that, but we often have not been able to point them in someone's direction, with the exception of a handful of people who become our regular commentators. We have been trying over time to expand that role of people openly living with HIV who feel equipped to be spokespeople, because it can also be pretty daunting, not just the issue, but media can be pretty daunting, and if you've got a difficult issue like criminalization, which I would say is our most difficult issue, always has been, it's even more daunting.

Reporters regularly referenced the importance of including quotations from people living with HIV in stories about HIV criminalization. A reporter named Rob understood personal narratives from people who live with HIV as a powerful journalistic device that helps to make the issue of HIV criminalization a newsworthy topic. As Rob described:

> When people are bogged down with x amount of people have been criminalized, 181 ... it's not a big number, let's not kid ourselves, that's not a lot of people. So, if you really want to talk about the hardship and the struggle that they've been through ... the situation those people are in before, and what happens to them inside, and what happens to them outside after, if they get out, it's you know, it changes it ... So, the personal narrative really sets it apart.

Other reporters described that speaking with people who have lived experience is an integral part of researching a news story. For instance, a journalist named Matthew explained that personal accounts "just bring the story home a little bit more." Another journalist, named Lindsay, related to spokespeople as essential resources for better understanding issues she is reporting on:

> Talking to people that are the most concerned, no matter what I'm writing about, is the most important part of a piece [news story]. Even though, in the end, in the article it's [quotes from spokespeople] a very, very small part of the article, when you write as a journalist, if you don't have the background, if you haven't spoken to people who are the most concerned, to me it's really hard to write ... to make it legitimate as a journalist, you just have to talk to people who live what you're talking about.

These remarks suggest that reporters require quotations from people with lived experience of HIV and/or criminalization in order to interrupt crime genre reports of HIV non-disclosure that typically objectify people living with HIV and write over the complexity of their experiences. It can, however, be a daunting exercise for one to share such personal experiences in the press. As Richard explained:

> People need to have a good grasp of the law and the legal system, because if you don't have a grounding in that and you get the question from the journalist and you answer incorrectly, then you're not necessarily being an effective advocate if you're misstating the law or you're, you're not sure how a certain thing came about ... if it's a live interview, especially on broadcast media, you don't really have a chance to sort that out, you've made the mistake and now it's done, there's no do-over. We want people to feel like they know what the basics of the law is and because the law

is still uncertain on some points and because there may be some room to manoeuvre on certain points like the viral load question where we're seeing different decisions emerging from different courts and we're trying to push it in a certain direction … In terms of how much of your own story are you willing to share? How much of it is it strategic to share? Or is it a matter of how you would deflect that question and take it back to your key message.

In this segment, the speaker identifies an astonishing range of skills that activists require in order to carry out work as spokespeople who can talk with reporters about this issue. First, spokespeople require a solid understanding of the criminal law as it pertains to HIV non-disclosure. As Richard indicates, this legal context is complex and continues to shift. One's capacity to speak to the intricacies of HIV criminalization also requires an understanding of medical science terminology, such as "the viral load question." In addition to these challenging characteristics of working as a spokesperson, people with lived experiences of HIV and/or criminalization must also strategically select and share aspects of their deeply personal story in a way that advances efforts to resist HIV criminalization. All the while, the pressure and stakes attached to activists' encounters with the media are high, as a spokesperson's work often occurs live, on air, and one's message is recorded and reprinted for the mass public to consume.

To support the presence of new spokespeople who have lived experiences of HIV and/or criminalization, the LN hosts media training workshops that are designed to equip participants with the tools that they require to be spokespeople against HIV criminalization. These workshops are important to acknowledge, because they are another means by which the LN links the relevancies of news production with a type of expert knowledge about HIV criminalization. Reporters continually expressed to the LN that it would be productive to interview spokespeople with lived experience, and the organization responded by working to support people who could speak from that position and connecting them to reporters. As Janet explained, "the next time journalists need a diversity of spokespeople I can be like, 'hey, we just did this training …'"

The central goal of the media training that the LN has developed is to build the practical skills of people living with HIV who are seeking ways to become public advocates against HIV criminalization. Following our interview, Janet shared with me the slide deck that she uses in training sessions. Much of the training focuses on strategies that advocates can use to craft and deliver their message in a news interview.

For example, participants are encouraged to build their story in three parts: begin with a brief summary of their experience, then place the story in a larger context of concerns about HIV criminalization, and end with a call to action. People with lived experiences of HIV and/or criminalization have adopted the conversational approach set out in the workshops, such as being brief and concise and staying on message. For instance, one spokesperson with lived experience of HIV and/or criminalization, named Steven, explained to me that during interviews he is always sure to:

> Not talk too long. Simple sentences with subject, predicate, and object. Don't try and be very nuanced, keep it really simple. Because as soon as you start to get into compound sentences and paragraphs and nuance, it's really easy for part of it to be lifted out, because that's the way they operate. Quotes can't be too long, and if the meaning of sentence three is dependent on sentence two and sentence two is dependent on sentence one, and you only get sentence three [included in the news article], game over. So, it has to be very simple, very short, and grammatically very straightforward.

The speaker's remarks are interesting for two reasons. First, because they provide valuable insight into the specific speech mechanics that advocates implement to have their message quoted coherently in news texts. In this example, the speaker describes that as he speaks to reporters, he anticipates how segments of his message will be isolated as quotations to be placed in a broader news text. His comments illustrate that one's work as a spokesperson not only necessitates knowledge of the context of HIV criminalization, it also requires a specialized way of structuring and delivering one's message in a way that aligns with reporters' news-writing practices.

Other activists that I interviewed who had experiences as spokespeople described similar tactics for ensuring their message lands in news articles. Tony, for example, explained, "I feel broad strokes don't paint as pretty a picture ... I tend to be a flowery talker, so one of the things that I know to do is to reel this in when I do media stuff." Likewise, Anne recounted:

> the whole process of editing and how they take the parts that they can use, not the parts that you actually wanted to get across ... you have to wonder if it's almost better to craft one or two statements and just leave it ... it is a challenge [to communicate] in a very small space [that news articles provide].

For these advocates, speaking as a spokesperson is largely an exercise in restricting and truncating their speech so that their intended message will flow into the final version of a news story.

A second significant feature of Steven's comments is that they show the organizing links that shape how one comes to be a spokesperson in the first place. The work that the LN does to mobilize its media expertise and train spokespeople is an important indicator that one's work as a spokesperson often takes place within a broad network of coordinated activity that includes HIV advocacy organizations, lawyers, communications specialists, activists and people with lived experiences of HIV who possess particular forms of specialized knowledge and expertise.

By inserting their messages about HIV criminalization into the mainstream press via the news interview, advocates work to disrupt the control that ideological and political authorities (such as police) exert in the media (301–2). Manuel Castells (2009a) argues that by using mainstream media to convey their messages, social movements increase their chances of enacting social change (302). However, Castells also warns that social movement actors' position as "alternative messengers come with servitude: they must adapt to the language of the media and to the forms of interaction in the communication networks" (302). While activists' accounts of their work in news interviews exemplify how they truncate their language to fit the forms and conventions of the news interview, the next sections of this chapter offer insight into how activists also expand the scope of their messages by producing news texts themselves.

Before moving on to discuss other types of media work that activists do, it is worth emphasizing the tremendous emotional labour that spokesperson work entails – especially for spokespeople with lived experiences of HIV and/or criminalization. Some advocates with lived experiences related to the opportunity to do spokesperson work as an enriching experience. For example, in the years since Kyle spent time in prison on criminal charges related to HIV non-disclosure, he has shared his story in the press in an effort to raise public awareness about the harsh penalties people living with HIV can face. He explained:

> As an activist, a lot of people will come to me as, you know, word of mouth. If you want to talk to someone who has lived experience and is willing to share his story ... you should find me. I'll talk to anyone, I don't have a problem sharing my story with anybody. The more I get to share my story, the more I get to heal.

As reporters' accounts illustrate, longer-form, more nuanced news stories about HIV criminalization are unlikely to be published without the work of spokespeople with lived experience, like Kyle. At the same time, it is also important to recognize that being a spokesperson on this issue can be a weighty experience. For example, Tanya is a person living with HIV who works with an AIDS service organization. She recounted that after an interview she did ran in the *Daily Report* she removed all of them from a newspaper box near her home:

> We have a store right by my house, the corner store, and they have the *Daily Report*, I actually took all the papers from the box and took them home with me. Because it's my neighbourhood, who knows what people see in it, and they could start talking, so I just took all the *Daily Reports*.

This story iterates that HIV organizations' media work should extend beyond media training workshops that help advocates insert their voices into the press to also include support following the publication of their experiences.

Text Production Work

Readers will recognize by now that there are tremendous challenges associated with advocates' efforts to shift the content of news reports about HIV criminalization. The work practices and routines of reporters who produce typical crime stories about HIV criminalization are deeply entrenched and fulfil news organizations' strategic goals. Furthermore, the accounts of HIV advocates in the previous section show that challenging mainstream news texts as a spokesperson is a highly complex exercise that requires one to respond to reporters' questions by condensing and mobilizing critiques of HIV criminalization. With this in mind, it is not surprising that advocates sometimes elect to bypass reporters altogether and produce their own news texts instead. One of the most visible ways that advocates produce news texts is by writing opinion editorial articles. As Janet from the Legal Network explains:

> An op-ed is a good venue for criminalization because criminalization in media relations terms is not a soundbite issue ... it's an issue that's a human rights issue, it's super important, but when you're getting edited down to like a two-sentence bite, it can easily be taken out of context, and that's happened to us ... So an op-ed allows us to fully develop the case so it makes a really good product for this issue in particular.

Janet's remarks call attention to some of the ways that opinion editorials work as productive vehicles for communicating activists' concerns about HIV criminalization. For one, whereas activists who respond to reporters' questions as spokespeople must learn to speak in a highly structured way and anticipate how reporters will select short segments of their message as quotations in a news article, opinion editorials provide space for activists to more fully convey the scope and tone of their messages. Activists can speak to the complexity and nuance of their perspectives on criminalization much more fully in the 900–1,200 words that opinion editorials make available than they can when one or two sentences from their interviews with reporters are inserted into news articles. Perhaps even more importantly, opinion editorials provide a way for HIV advocates to be the sole speaker in a news text. This allows them to exercise much greater control over their message than occasions when they are interviewed as spokespeople, only to have reporters position their voices alongside authorities such as police, public health officers, and Crown attorneys.

I came to better appreciate the way that opinion editorial articles can meaningfully reshape news discourse about HIV criminalization during my interview with Diane. Diane is the executive director of a small ASO in a town I'll call Greenville. In the summer of 2017, a young man in Greenville was arrested and charged with multiple counts of aggregated sexual assault. Greenville police alleged that he had unprotected sex without disclosing his HIV-positive status. Diane learned of the criminal charge when local media agencies circulated a police news release that included the young man's photo, age, details about when the incidents occurred, reference to the online dating sites he used, and encouraged anyone who believed they may have "been exposed" to seek medical attention. Almost right away, Diane began to see the stigmatizing effects of crime genre reporting play out on social media. As she described,

> posting the picture … in all these places is inflammatory and likely not helpful in this situation and it's sparking a lot of debate on social media … there's this stuff happening in media, social media, where all those early, awful, awful things that came up, and someone had posted, they posted things like people living with HIV should have it branded on their forehead so we all know.

The media coverage of this case, and the ensuing vitriol that spread on social media, call to mind the most sensational and stigmatizing types of representations of HIV. What is striking about the case in Greenville, however, is the way that Diane produced opinion editorial texts that interrupted the crime genre narrative and even transformed how knowledge about HIV non-disclosure is produced and disseminated in Greenville.

In an effort to learn more about how Diane responded to the infamous news coverage of the Greenville case, I arranged to drive to the town and meet with her at the ASO. The agency reminded me of the small ASO that I worked at when I first began working in the field of HIV as an education outreach coordinator in 2010. I was greeted warmly by a volunteer who was working at the front desk, and I sat in the waiting area as people passed by to see support workers, to take part in volunteer-run programs, and to collect harm-reduction supplies. Diane began our conversation by explaining some of the particular challenges the ASO currently faces:

> Our work has focused on people living with HIV, people affected by HIV, people at risk of HIV, and in particular using injection drugs ... We're a small organization, we've never been more than ten staff with a huge area [to serve] ... The work now, the number of people who are living with HIV who come to our ASO for service is small compared to the number of people who use injection drugs because we run the needle exchange harm-reduction program. Now naloxone and overdose prevention training, and that's eating us alive and turning us into a crisis-based organization, so we actually don't have the infrastructure to do the work that we want to be able to do. We want to be able to respond more effectively to the queer community. We do a tremendous amount of training, anti-homophobia, positive space training, in the four counties, and then we lost federal funding, so we lost the capacity to do some of that.

The executive director describes that the work of the small staff and volunteers at the ASO is mostly about responding to crisis, and the challenging work that they do is exacerbated by funding cuts. In such a context, they do not have the capacity to carry out all of the initiatives that they recognize are necessary to meet the needs of the community that they serve and, of course, do not have ample resources or specialized media expertise to devote to public relations activities.

Although the ASO was already over-extended in many ways when the news story started to circulate in 2017, Diane initiated a response almost right away. Her first step was to contact local media agencies and request that they pull the police news release from their news websites. Most news agencies declined because the news story was considered a matter of public safety. As Diane explains, "we were told by radio and TV that they couldn't pull the news release down because it was a public safety message from the Chief of Police and so they're bound at a policy level to [publish them]." This response from media organizations is interesting because it helps to show the extent to which news content is coordinated by texts and information that police publish. In an effort to decouple police messages about public safety from popular understandings of HIV non-disclosure, Diane and the ASO produced news texts that were intended to amplify advocates' concerns about HIV criminalization.

Diane explained, "where we saw our particular role was, it wasn't to talk about that particular case, it was to broaden the conversation, bring it back to [the problems with] criminalization." After media organizations refused to remove the police press release from their sites, the ASO "asked Greenville police if they would, we let them know we were working on a statement, and they agreed to post it on their site, directly below the chief's public safety warning."

In addition to the addendum to the news articles, the ASO also published a lengthier opinion editorial article. The editorial emphasized concerns about how the criminal law responds to non-disclosure and called for all legal and policy responses to HIV to be based on the best available evidence and in line with the objectives of HIV prevention, care, treatment, and respect for human rights.

The articles that Diane's organization crafted help to show how a stable and consistent response to stigmatizing news coverage is put together. Although Diane is not a professional researcher or legal expert, the work of community-based HIV legal advocacy organizations makes it possible for Diane to write in the way that she did. Community-based legal advocacy organizations, such as the LN, publish documents that synthesize key critiques of HIV criminalization, such as calls for legal responses to be brought in-line with scientific evidence about HIV transmission, as well as reminders that most people living with HIV disclose their status and that safer sex is a shared responsibility (Canadian HIV/ AIDS Legal Network 2014; Hastings, Kazatchkine, and Mykhalovskiy 2017). In addition to publishing documents, legal experts also regularly deliver workshops at ASOs across the province. For example, during our interview, Diane described that one of her sources for learning about how to engage with media on the issue of HIV criminalization was a presentation that Ryan Peck, the director of the HIV/AIDS Legal Clinic of Ontario, had delivered in Greenville. When I spoke to Ryan, he explained, "we end up speaking all around the province about this ... we do lots of workshops, like hundreds and hundreds. So, over the last ten or eleven years ... I've probably ran 350, 400 speaking engagements, a lot of them on this issue [of HIV criminalization]." This type of training is an important part of the broader organized response to stigmatizing news stories and helps to support interventions like Diane's.

The news texts that the ASO produced are discursively significant, in that they countered the crime genre reports that spur stigma and hostility towards people living with HIV. Perhaps even more significantly, the news texts that the ASO authored were the basis for dialogue with police that brought about material changes to how knowledge about HIV is produced in Greenville. As Diane described, following the publication of their messages the ASO asked Greenville police:

> "If you're going to lay more charges, or if you ever charge someone with aggravated sexual assault for not disclosing their HIV status, can you give us a couple of hours before you go ahead with your public warning?" They granted that [request] ... so that's fantastic ... I think that police here had a significant learning, and I think it would be safe for me to say that if another, if a similar situation would arise in Greenville again, the current staff at Greenville Police would handle it differently.

I like to think of this quote as a way to acknowledge how the response to crime genre reports of HIV criminalization is put together. Diane's account of the ASO's media intervention shows that HIV advocates' presence in the news media does not always take the form of reporters from major newspapers with national circulation calling upon public relations experts who work for widely recognized NGOs. Influential media interventions are also the product of work done by HIV service providers who are highly attentive and responsive to ways that knowledge about HIV criminalization is produced and circulated, and coordinate responses to media off the side of their desk while also providing front-line responses to HIV.

At the same time, the type of intervention Janet described in the previous section and the response that Diane illustrates in this section can both be understood as efforts to coordinate the knowledge of HIV advocates with the relevancies of news media production. As Diane described, one of the reasons that the opinion editorial made sense as a format is because "we realized that in a small community the media need to be our partners and that we can feed them information and work with them in a way that gives them what they're looking for." In this case, the texts she wrote summarize critiques of HIV criminalization that are well known among HIV advocates and fit them into the format of an opinion editorial article so that they can circulate as a news text. What her activities accomplish is the coordination of advocates' knowledge about HIV criminalization with the routines and structure of news production.

Creating Texts for News Production

Diane's account of her work shows how advocates vie to interrupt crime genre reports about HIV criminal cases by producing news texts that are inscribed with their concerns and critiques of HIV criminalization. In this section, I want to illustrate another type of text production work that targets the mainstream news. Here, I reflect on my experiences as a researcher who has published documents that are not news texts in and of themselves but are intended to shape how journalists report on HIV non-disclosure. I came to understand how my research activities on these projects are hooked into a network of professional knowledge and the expertise of those who work to end HIV criminalization during my interview with a reporter named James.

James covers legal issues for a large newspaper called the *Daily Post*. I met with James to learn more about how he had constructed a recent news article about HIV non-disclosure in Canada. The article was not a standard crime story about HIV criminalization. Instead, it foregrounded activists' voices, included quotations from someone with lived experience of HIV criminalization, and provided readers with important context about how the criminal law is used to respond to HIV non-disclosure in Canada. His article exemplifies the sort of contextualized, thoughtful, nuanced reporting that HIV advocates have been calling for. As we sat across from each other on well-worn, but comfortable couches near his desk in a corner of the newsroom, James described that a particular factsheet published by the Canadian HIV/AIDS Legal Network had been helpful for his news writing. As a co-author of that report, it was exciting for me to hear that James had taken it up in his newswork:

> I just find it really helpful, certainly a lot of information ... I put into my own story, obviously sourcing where it came from ... So, it's really easy to look at that and it gives you a great idea of what the issues are right now and who's being affected in terms of ethnicity, sexual orientation, because some of it's broken down like that, which is really helpful ... it's based on actual, hard data, hard numbers.

As James described the structure of the document and recounted the data in the report, I did not get the sense that he knew that I had co-authored it (along with an academic researcher and a lawyer who

works at the HIV Legal Network). It was a somewhat strange experience to have him carefully explain to me that "at least 184 people in 200
cases have been charged in relation to HIV non-disclosure since 1989"
as a straightforward statement of fact. As the reporter recounted the statistic, it was as if our work as researchers, and the research process that
we carried out to produce that statement, had been forgotten. Reflecting
on the interview now, I understand that this sort of "forgetting" of the
originating researchers and research activities is significant because it
signals that research findings have attained factual status (Latour and
Woolgar 1986; D.E. Smith 1990).

When one reads a factual statement in James's news article (such
as "at least 184 people in 200 cases have been charged in relation
to HIV non-disclosure since 1989"), the reader of the news text is
not prompted to consider our lengthy meetings at legal offices sur-
rounded by stacks of folders brimming with legal documents, or the
hours we spent constructing databases to record and sort information about cases, or the time I spent entering data into Excel files, or
of the multiple drafts, edits, and versions that the authors produced
prior to publishing – for the news reader "what remains is only the
text, which aims at being read as 'what actually happened/what is'"
(D.E. Smith 1990, 79). I reflect on how my co-authors and I produced
a factual account of HIV criminalization, becuase the story of how
data moved from digital and hard-copy folders held by lawyers and
ASO workers, to the desk where I work in my apartment, to a report
we published, to the desk of James and other reporters, to news
texts that we read, and then back to my during my interview with
James ...

At the time I started to work on the factsheet with the LN, I had
recently co-authored and published an analysis of the unequal way that
HIV criminal non-disclosure cases have been covered in mainstream
newspapers ("'Callous, Cold and Deliberately Duplicitous': Racialization, Immigration and the Representation of HIV Criminalization in
Canadian Mainstream Newspapers"). The media study was funded by
a grant from the Canadian Institutes of Health Research (CIHR) Centre
for Social Research in HIV Prevention. This funding initiative encour-
ages a particular type of research partnership between community
leaders and academic researchers and supports "research that will lead
to practical and useful outcomes that will directly benefit the community" (Canadian Institutes of Health Research 2018). In this instance,
our project was an attempt to produce a type of scholarship that would
contribute to an evidentiary response to the concerns expressed by African, Caribbean, and Black activists; people living with HIV; and ASOs

that African, Caribbean, and Black people living with HIV are negatively portrayed and overrepresented in Canadian newspaper stories about HIV non-disclosure (Mykhalovskiy et al. 2016, 5).

One of the important outcomes of the media analysis was that it publicized the skewed pattern of news stories and the stigmatizing tone of crime story reporting about HIV criminal non-disclosure cases. In some instances, our analysis of the news discourse of HIV criminalization became the focus of news stories themselves, with headlines such as "Media Accused of Racism in Reporting HIV-related Crime" (Keung 2016), "Canadian News Coverage of HIV Assaults Proven to be Racist" (Easton 2016), and "New Report Suggests Racism in Canadian Newspaper Articles About HIV" (Goh 2017). Having helped to establish a stable empirical foundation to bolster activists' claims that Canadian newspapers are a source of profoundly stigmatizing representations of people living with HIV, I was starting to think about how to move from producing analyses of news content to producing research that could help to re-shape news content.

Around that time, I was approached by a policy analyst from the LN who asked if I would be interested in co-authoring a factsheet that would update information on the outcomes of HIV non-disclosure cases and test advocates' inclination that the Supreme Court of Canada's decision in 2012 had harshened the legal obligation to disclose one's HIV-positive status. I was keen to contribute to the production of a report that could be used in advocacy efforts to end HIV criminalization, and I also related to this research project as a way to intervene in reporters' newswork processes. As the analyst from the LN explained, the document was to be structured upon the data that reporters requested from the organization most often:

> I mean journalists, they want numbers, they want, every time you do an interview, they ask how many people have been charged? How many cases involve transmission? How many cases resulted in conviction? They want those numbers.

Our sense was that if statistical data that illustrated the concerning patterns and trends of HIV criminalization were made visible and easily accessible to reporters, it could provide the basis upon which they could produce news stories that diverged from typical crime stories. Scholars of governmentality might explain our efforts to represent the social phenomenon of HIV criminalization in statistical terms as an exercise in "describing a world such that it is amenable to having certain things done to it" (Miller and Rose 1990, 7). Typically studies of governmentality call attention to ways that quantitative methods and statistical representation make the governance of social life possible (Latour 1987; Porter 1995).

As Miller and Rose write,

> Describing a world such that it is amenable to having certain things done to it involves inscribing reality into the calculations through a range of material and rather mundane techniques (Rose 1988; Latour 1986). This form enables the pertinent features of the domain – types of goods, investments, ages of person, health, criminality, etc. to literally be re-presented in the place where decisions are to be made about them (the manager's office, the war room, the case conference and so forth). (Miller and Rose 1990, 7).

Analyses of governmentality consider the ways that quantitative methods permit reasoned, highly rule-bound, or officially sanctioned modes of measurement (Porter 1995, 5–6). However, our aim in producing the statistical factsheet (comprising quantification and visual displays of numerical information about HIV criminalization) was to make the injustice of HIV criminalization visible to reporters in a way that moved activists' critiques of HIV criminalization into the newsroom, and subsequently into news texts. Ultimately, our goal was to represent HIV criminalization as a problem that needed to be addressed urgently and to encourage widespread social and political mobilization.

I understand the research process of producing the numbers that reporters want as an intricate exercise in coordinating a range of expert knowledge about HIV criminalization. This process started with the Legal Network reaching out and partnering with myself and another academic researcher – and then our research work activities were about accessing and gathering various types of knowledge that professionals working in the field of HIV advocacy had produced or had access to. This included adding information to a database of criminal trials related to HIV non-disclosure cases that an academic researcher and a lawyer had last updated in 2012. We also met with lawyers (who referenced their legal files and documents and sometimes consulted with other lawyers and HIV service providers) and reviewed news articles. Once the data was collected, we collaborated on activities to produce texts and publish our findings. We constructed tables that illustrated our key findings, wrote analytic descriptions of the patterns we observed in our data, and (following numerous drafts, edits, meetings, and emails among the authors) published reports that produced a factual account of how the criminal law is used to respond to HIV non-disclosure in Canada.

This wide range of research and writing activities was coordinated by an effort to produce factual accounts of HIV criminalization and to publish them in an accessible format, "the factsheet," that corresponded to reporters' fast-paced and text-based work routines. As one HIV legal advocate who we consulted on the project described:

> We know they're [reporters are] totally time stretched, and so it's hard for them to devote the time to do the really careful thinking and diving in depth into the issue, because they just don't have the time, which is a terrible situation to be in, but if we can give them like, "here's a factsheet that in two pages gives you the number of prosecutions, some commentary about the problems with what leads to the prosecutions, and some specific things that we say should be done to address that problem, like prosecutorial guidelines, for example, or a moratorium until guidelines are developed," those are easy pieces for them for, "okay, that's what advocates are saying about this, and I know now that there have been 185 cases and half of them have been in Ontario, those are easy facts for me to just copy and paste into an article."

Producing texts that are inscribed with advocates' critiques and concerns expressed as what James recognized as "hard data, hard numbers" makes critiques and concerns about HIV criminalization available to reporters in a form that they can efficiently transfer into a news article. Statistical data is known to have purchase in news discourse and operate in news stories as a way to establish truth and facticity. As Teun van Dijk writes:

> [T]he rhetoric of news discourse forcefully suggests truthfulness by the implied exactness of precise numbers. This is one of the reasons why news discourse abounds with numerical indications of many kinds ... Few rhetorical ploys more convincingly suggest truthfulness than these number games ... Again, it is not so much the precision of the numbers that is relevant but rather the fact that numbers are given at all ... They are predominantly meant as signals of precision and hence truthfulness. (van Dijk 1988, 87–8).

In the months following the publication of our report, we saw data from the factsheet appear in news texts. In some news articles, data from our report interrupted straightforward crime reporting by providing important context about HIV criminalization, expressed as plainspoken statements of fact.[3] We were especially encouraged by news stories that drew on data from the report as a way to produce HIV criminalization as a pressing social justice concern and to mobilize critiques of how the criminal law is used to respond HIV non-disclosure in Canada. For example, news articles included data from the factsheet in order to highlight that the criminal law is out of step with current science on HIV transmission,[4] and that criminal justice sentences in cases of HIV non-disclosure are exceptionally punitive.[5] These news articles suggest that our efforts to coordinate knowledge and the expertise of HIV advocates that was spread across universities, NGOs, and legal offices into a single factsheet that fit the relevancies of news production processes, has been an effective way to support the publication of news stories that diverge from crime stories and amplify HIV advocates' critiques of criminalization.

The traction that numerical data from our report gained in news reports exemplifies a specific way that social movements can create a counter-discourse. In particular, this experience illustrates the importance of numbers in grounding a factual discourse that can shape people's understanding of injustices that are linked to HIV criminalization. As Mary Poovey (1998, 5) writes, numbers connote "transparency and impartiality that have made them so perfectly suited to the epistemological work performed by the modern fact." In this instance, the factual counter-discourse that we mobilized was made possible by a particular type of collaborative research that the HIV community has

---

3 For example: "the Canadian HIV/AIDS Legal Network has counted at least 180 people charged for offences related to HIV non-disclosure in Canada since 1989" (J. Turner 2014, 4); "At least 180 people charged for HIV non-disclosure since 1989, Canadian HIV/AIDS Legal Network says" (Canadian Press 2017); "Ontario leads in the number of people charged with HIV status non-disclosure and 180 people have been charged across the country, Jonathan Valelly of Queers Crash the Beat said at the protest" (Beeston 2017).

4 "There have been 210 cases since 1989 in Canada in which the HIV status of the person charged was a central issue, according to the Canadian HIV/AIDS Legal Network. In most of those cases, there was little or no chance of the virus being transmitted because of condom use, low viral load or low-risk activities such as oral sex. Yet the majority resulted in convictions" (Picard 2018).

5 "According to the Canadian HIV/AIDS Legal Network, the conviction rate for HIV non-disclosure is higher than the conviction rate for sexual assault in Canada, at 70 per cent and 24 per cent, respectively. This suggests that the courts are interpreting the mere possibility of transmitting HIV as more dangerous than sexual assault – despite the fact HIV is no longer a death sentence and that in most of these cases, HIV wasn't transmitted" (Bogosavljevic and Kilty 2017, A7).

been promoting for decades (Trussler and Marchand 2005). Funding mechanisms encourage and support connections between university-based researchers (such as myself and co-author Eric Mykhalovskiy) and those who work at HIV organizations (such as co-author Cecile Kazatchkine from the HIV Legal Network) that are designed to inform responses to HIV.

Relational Work

The final type of work activity that advocates regularly described during interviews had to do with building relationships with reporters to facilitate their concerns about HIV criminalization making it into news reports. This sort of work often occurred early in the criminal justice processing of a criminal HIV non-disclosure case. As Richard described, one of the LN's first steps is to:

> reach out to some news reporters who will cover the issue, because they might have covered it in the past for their local media, or just because they have covered it in the past for their local media, we think if it's not on their radar, if we put it on their radar they might actually write something useful.

Richard's comments are interesting because they reinforce the idea that news stories about HIV criminalization that include advocates' voices do not "just happen." Instead, they are the product of advocates' efforts to anticipate newsworthy events related to HIV non-disclosure, to have a sense of which reporters are most likely to write favourable reports of the event, and to maintain relationships with those reporters that allow advocates to connect them to these newsworthy items. Janet Butler-McPhee, the communications director, described her efforts to reach out to reporters and encourage them to write about HIV criminalization as a type of extended media relations work:

> Well, people think of media relations as hitting send on a press release, but I think the real importance of media relations is understanding [reporters are] also trying to do a job and they're trying to do it well. And their job isn't necessarily to advocate for your cause ... but they're under time pressures too, they want a great story ... So it's not just calling them when you need something from them. I just met with one of the reporters I know, I was just like, "hey, what's your interest?" and I met with the *Daily Gazette* at the same time ... both basically taking

notes on what each other needed, and then the reporter explained, "you know, we tend to have a lot of trouble filling the Sunday online spot ... getting content is really hard because people want it to appear on Monday morning's paper in print." So I thought, "oh, if I can find some things, ideas that could move the story further" ... *News Centre* ended up writing a piece that got picked up about criminalization ... and that was because we orchestrated that.

In a previous section of this chapter, we learned that Janet conceptualizes news interviews as a style of dance. Here, we can see that the communications director's rhythm with reporters also takes the form of "orchestrating" the production of news stories that are structured upon the LN's critiques and concerns about HIV criminalization. Janet accomplishes this by coming to understand the gaps in news organizations' production processes and routines, and identifying ways to fill those openings with content about advocates' efforts to end HIV criminalization. This style of relational work that Janet describes helps to insert the LN's concerns about HIV and the criminal law into public discourse. At the same time, reporters benefit from gaining access to a newsworthy story and from the support of advocates (like Janet) who help facilitate quick, efficient, and consistent news production. One reporter I interviewed described how Janet supported her reporting on HIV criminalization:

She asked me out for coffee, and we just had a chat about what they do, what I do, how we can sort of help each other out. They had mentioned, and I had actually, it was so below the radar and so lacking in hoopla and bells and whistles that I had missed the statement from the Minister on World AIDS Day mentioning that she'd be working on fixing the problem [of HIV criminalization], I was really intrigued by that. I guess it was either that week or the next week when I had some time that I had said to my editor, "you know, this has happened now a couple of weeks ago, but no one's really written about it yet, in the mainstream press anyway." I think it's a big deal, I know a lot of people care about it, so she said go for it. That's how I wrote my first story on this issue.

In this instance, Janet called the reporter's attention to an important landmark in activists' efforts to reform HIV criminalization. The statement from former Justice Minister and Attorney General Jody Wilson-Raybould on World AIDS Day 2017 was widely recognized as a significant breakthrough because the Minister echoed perspectives that advocates had voiced for years, including concerns about ways that HIV criminalization discourages people from being tested for HIV. If not for the relationship that Janet formed with the journalist, this important milestone in advocates' efforts might have gone unreported and unnoticed. However, Janet was able to help the reporter recognize that this issue is "a big deal" and that "a lot of people care about it."

I understand Janet's account of her work to cultivate relationships with reporters as another example of how advocates try to shape news coverage of HIV criminalization by coordinating their knowledge and expertise with news production processes and routines. It would be understandable for one who reads Janet's account of her rapport with the press (or Diane's account of crafting opinion editorial articles, or my reflections on how co-authors and I produced factual accounts for reporters to draw on) to conclude that advocates can efficiently insert their messages into the mainstream news through a variety of straightforward work activities. However, by beginning analysis with the experiences of HIV advocates who are positioned in different HIV advocacy organizations, we learn that while the possibility of coordinating advocacy work with the relevancies of journalism exists, it is not equally available to everyone.

In different locations of the everyday world of HIV advocacy, there is a noticeable lack of connection between reporters and HIV advocates. I came to understand this disparity during an interview with Naomi. Naomi is the executive director of a community health centre that specializes in providing primary health care for racialized people living with HIV. Most of the other HIV advocates whom I interviewed work with organizations that are racialized as mainly (though not entirely) white and are involved in issues around racialization and anti-racism by supporting refugees and people who have migrated living with HIV; supporting legal reforms to protect the health and safety of LGBTQ2+ people in Caribbean countries; and collaborating with Indigenous communities to respond to HIV. Naomi is one of the only interviewees who works for an organization that represents racialized communities exclusively.

As the director of the organization, she is responsible for managing the staff, securing funding, overseeing the organization's finances, as well as being "the front-face of the organization, I'm the person out in public or in the media speaking on behalf of the organization and promoting our agenda." In some ways, Naomi faces challenges that are similar to those that Diane confronts at the ASO. Both of their organizations provide front-line HIV services with limited resources, and both executive directors work to engage with the media without the resources or media expertise that are available to some larger NGOs.

Naomi explained that her approach to engaging with media is informed by the deeply troubling way that the press has covered HIV criminalization and, in particular, HIV criminal cases that involve African, Caribbean, and Black defendants throughout her twenty-five years working in this field of HIV. She described:

> I started in this work twenty-five years ago, so I kind of caught the beginning of that media coverage for African populations in particular. So, the C.S case for me is where it starts. It's just how that got sensationalized and there hasn't been a disruption to that narrative. It just feeds into anti-Black racism, anti-immigrant sentiments, all of that. So, all I've seen is how racialized women, Indigenous women get caught up in that narrative. Right? So, they just get the female version of that narrative. How racialized women often get sexualized, over-sexualized, and described as going to put the Canadian public in danger.

Naomi's remarks articulate the types of concerns that HIV advocates, particularly African, Caribbean, and Black advocates, have long been expressing about news coverage of HIV criminalization. The executive director's comments trace a lineage of deeply troubling news coverage that spans her entire career. The case of C.S that she mentions began in 1991 and was the first HIV non-disclosure case to receive widespread press coverage. A defining characteristic of news reports about C.S was how they relied on age-old tropes of dangerous Black masculinity and emphasized his immigration to Canada from Uganda in order to represent him as a dangerous, racialized Other (Mykhalovskiy et al. 2021b). As Naomi identifies, this type of sensational, racializing narrative of HIV criminalization started with coverage of the C.S case in 1991 and has largely remained stable in the decades since.

The executive director explained that the deeply entrenched crime genre narrative about HIV criminalization informs the way that she engages (or does not engage) with the mainstream press. She described her interaction with reporters as "very, very controlled." For Naomi, this means:

> not doing print [interviews] unless we're going to get the transcript back so that we can, you know, all those kinds of things that maybe other people don't, they have a different experience with the media and they trust it and they see it as way to promote their organization. And for us, we don't use the media to promote our organization … We don't give commentary on live issues. So, you won't see like, something happens and, then you know how they, "can you comment on this thing," right? We don't do that.

> There's a lot of fear because the thing is our reputation with our communities that we serve is crucial, and we're talking about criminalization and the media has probably added the most to the stigma that the Black community has experienced. So, you don't also want to be seen as siding with a medium that has not been good to this particular community.

In this quotation, the speaker starts to bring into view how race organizes the social relations of mainstream media. Naomi's remarks show that the long lineage of racist and stigmatizing news coverage mean that community-based organizations are highly reluctant to connect with the press, seek out media attention, or respond to requests for interviews. Because these social relations position her organization in relation to media in this way, Naomi does particular types of media work. Along with the typical challenges that come with attempting to disrupt the stable and consistent crime genre narrative (that have been displayed in this chapter) Naomi also describes that she has to work to establish trust and, in some cases, disconnect from mainstream media in order to protect and maintain the reputation that her organization has with racialized people living with HIV. While other advocates I spoke with in this chapter described their efforts to align their organization's work with the press, Naomi explained that her organization has largely abandoned the standard repertoire of media relations activities:

> I think we gave up a long time ago trying to do press releases. I remember spending a lot of time sending out press releases on, you know, these great stories or things you're working on or programs you're developing, there's no bite. But when there's something controversial where we need to alert the rest of Canada of this bizarre practice or this barbaric practice or this threat to our Canadianness, then the phone is ringing off the hook ... I mean it's just a lot of frustration of trying to get messages out. I remember one major outlet saying to us, it was our anniversary so we're like oh this is fantastic, this organization has been around twenty years, people are going to come cover this event. And the newscaster saying, "unless someone gets killed or is dead at that event, we're not coming." And I'm like really? And she's like, "no, that's what we want to know from your community. That's what will get you on the news." She was being very honest, it was somebody that I know, she's a major broadcaster and she was just being very honest, that's the reality of the situation.

This disquieting account from Naomi illustrates how race operates institutionally in ways that create tensions between an ASO that represents African, Caribbean, and Black people and the mainstream media. Because the press continues to be an exceedingly marginalizing space for Naomi as she tries to publicize her organization's activities, the organization has largely jettisoned the mainstream news altogether:

> But yeah, I think that's when we realized, wait a minute, we can disrupt this story ourselves. We can produce our own messaging and our own material, we didn't have social media back then, but now that we do, not relying on mainstream media to get [be more] positive, what you can do now is disrupt their messages with your alternative messages.

The speaker's comments are important because they show that interventions in standard crime genre stories about HIV criminalization are not always about connecting the work of advocates with the work of journalists. In some situations, such as the one that Naomi describes, advocates purposefully disconnect from the mainstream press. In this case, the community organization rarely seeks the attention of news outlets and prefers to utilize social media and other digital spaces in order to produce a counter-discourse (Feltwell et al. 2017, 350). For example, the executive director explained that a documentary that the organization produced rejects common racializing tropes and stereotypes that circulate in standard, sensational crime stories of HIV criminalization. In place of the short crime reports that objectify people living with HIV, the documentary offers a long-form look at "women for a year of their lives, like sharing their lives for a year, what it really feels like to live with HIV, no one had seen that before." The documentary offers a perspective of the lives of racialized women who live with HIV that is not typically available to readers of mainstream news, and it has been a tremendously successful endeavour. Naomi explained that more than 15,000 copies have been distributed worldwide, and it continues to be an important online resource for the organization.

Media texts, such as the documentary and social media activity, can be understood as a powerful form of opposition to a mainstream press that has consistently disparaged, marginalized, and ignored the experiences of racialized women living with HIV. By producing their own media messages online, via social media, and through documentary films, the organization joins a long lineage of HIV activists who have produced their own media content in order to speak for themselves and combat the messages of those who speak for and about them. When communities who are normally spoken for and spoken about speak for themselves, they create a counter-discourse, which is an act of resistance to power oppressing them (Feltwell et al. 2017, 350; Foucault 1970; Moussa and Scapp 1996).

More specifically, the organization's media work might be understood as an important example of "Black counter-discourse" that activists produce to assert an alternative perspective that challenges dominant discourse, centre Black experiences, focus on issues most salient to Black audiences, and critique white-dominated institutions (Browne, Deckard, and Rodriguez 2016, 521; Fraser 1990). While studies of social movement interactions with mainstream media referenced in this chapter recognize how activists strategically insert their messages into public space via the mainstream press, critical race scholars remind us that access to such a public space is not equal and is shaped by intersections of race, class, gender, and sexuality (Pough 2004, 16). Although social media far from remedies this issue of universal accessibility to the public sphere, there is an emerging field of research that understands social media as a public sphere where Black activists effectively intervene in public discourse (Gallagher et al. 2018). The counter-discourse that Naomi's organization produces offers another important example of how Black activists skilfully assert power over public discourse by creating a public space to express their experiences and viewpoints (Carney 2016, 198).

It is important to recognize the ways that Naomi's organization skilfully mobilizes its expert knowledge in order to engage with media in a way that fits the needs of the communities that it serves. It is, of course, a tremendous triumph to oppose the long lineage of deeply troubling representations of HIV criminal non-disclosure cases that include African, Caribbean, and Black people and people who are newcomers to Canada. And the organization's ability to produce its own media initiatives, such as the documentary, is certainly worthy of celebration, especially considering that they do this media work not as a public relations firm or a research-based NGO, but as a front-line HIV service agency, navigating the day-to-day challenges that work entails.

While acknowledging and applauding the counter-narrative that Naomi's organization produces, it is important not to view their struggle with media as a sentimental triumph. Given the ongoing overrepresentation of African, Caribbean, and Black defendants in newspaper coverage of HIV non-disclosure criminal cases, organizations that represent these communities have an important and unique role to play in developing and mobilizing forms of counter-discourse. However, as the experiences of advocates in this chapter bring into view, producing a consistent and coherent discourse to oppose HIV criminalization is complex, resource-intensive work. And so, the efforts of ASOs and other organizations that are part of African, Caribbean, and Black communities and work with African, Caribbean, and Black people, deserve and require collective, widespread support from across organizations that oppose HIV criminalization.

Chapter Five

Conclusion

In closing, I return to the book's two overarching narratives: one part of this book traces the social organization of knowledge about HIV criminalization. This study recognizes the press as an important aspect of a broad complex of social relations that sustain HIV criminalization and offers an account of how stigmatizing news stories about the topic are produced and circulated. By making visible the social relations of news production about HIV criminalization, I hope to offer a basis for activist interventions into objectifying and stigmatizing crime genre stories about HIV criminalization. Another part of this book is an empirical study of how the news media ecosystem is put together, with particular attention to how the newswork that journalists do in newsrooms is hooked into and made possible by the work that others are doing in disparate sites. More specifically, this IE underscores the extent to which writing for digital news is about activating digital source texts and processing them into news texts as quickly and efficiently as possible. As I argued in the introduction, this social organization of writing for digital news sets reporters up to produce sensational news articles.

This book is a study of overlapping social relations across three empirical sites. It examines how news content about HIV criminalization is produced and reproduced through the coordinated (and also sometimes purposefully disjointed) work of newsmakers, police, and HIV advocates.

In chapter 2, I began by looking closely at what journalists do to produce a news article. Interviews with newsmakers helped to show the enormous pressure that they face to consistently produce online news content that will attract "clicks," "likes," and "shares" from online news readers. I argued that because the social organization of digital news production facilitates the production of sensational accounts of news, it should perhaps not come as a surprise that reports of HIV criminalization are consistently structured as a genre of sensational crime stories. In chapter 3, I studied how reporters' everyday newswork is linked to the work of those whom they rely on as sources of news stories. When talking to reporters about the newswork activities that they accomplished to produce news stories about HIV criminalization, they regularly described that their news texts were heavily based on police news release documents. My central argument in chapter 3 is that police news release texts accommodate the flow of police information and reasoning into the mainstream press and allow the police's construction of crime, public safety, risk, and security to be active in mainstream news accounts of HIV criminalization. Finally, my attention in chapter 4 is devoted to the work that HIV advocates do to intervene in mainstream news discourse and interrupt crime genre accounts of criminal HIV non-disclosure cases. Advocates' descriptions of their media work show that news discourse is not univocal and display how social movements produce counter-discourse by adding their messages and critiques of HIV criminalization into news texts. This type of media work can re-shape public knowledge of HIV criminalization in important ways.

Limitations

Before reflecting on what this project might teach us about IE, HIV criminalization, and mainstream media discourse, I want to identify some of the limits to this project. There are a number of limitations that have to do with ethnographic access to empirical sites. For example, at the outset of my project, my hope was that I would be afforded opportunities to shadow reporters for extended periods of time and follow them over the course of a number of complete workdays. This would allow me to ethnographically observe their newswork in action and enable me to foster a richer and more complete description of how reporters do the work of pitching stories to editors, deciding which stories to report on, contacting and interviewing sources, writing up news stories, sending news articles to web editors, and updating news articles. While I obviously was not hoping for new criminal charges related to HIV non-disclosure to be laid while I was conducting fieldwork, had one emerged while I was conducting this type of shadowing, I may have also gained important insights into how reporters cover HIV criminal non-disclosure cases from beginning to end. As it turns out, it was challenging to locate reporters who had time to be research participants amid their hectic work schedules and often irregular hours. Those who did agree to participate in this study understandably could not commit to being available for longer than interviews that lasted about an hour. Furthermore, because of concerns about confidentiality and in the interest of convenience, reporters often preferred to meet outside of their workplace and to hold interviews at their local coffee spot. In light of these limitations related to ethnographic access that would have allowed me to observe more of reporters' newswork, I relied on reporters' detailed descriptions of their work and fieldnotes from occasions when I was able to hold interviews in newsrooms.

Another limitation that relates to ethnographic access has to do with interviewing police. The interface between reporters' newswork and the work of police communications departments is an important part of this book; however, as I detail in chapter 3, interviewing police officers or gaining any sort of ethnographic access to police work was an arduous exercise. Meanwhile, the one interview that I was able to secure with a member of a police force was a less than comfortable experience. This project would have benefited from a deeper empirical account of how police communications departments do their work. This type of institutional ethnographic research could bring into view how a police officer decides to bring a particular case to a communications department, the ways that communications departments make decisions about which cases to publish news releases about (or decide to not publish news releases), and what it looks like when a communications department fields questions from reporters who are writing crime genre stories. While it is somewhat disappointing to think about what could have been had I been able to gain greater access to observe police communications work, I relate to the barriers that blocked my ethnographic access to police as an interesting research finding in and of itself. The relative protection from critical, empirical analysis that police authorities seem to enjoy speaks to one way that police uphold inequitable social relations.

Finally, there are limitations that have to do with the scope of this inquiry. The types of limitations that are present in this study are common among studies of mainstream news (Seale 2003). For one, this book addresses the production of news stories about HIV criminalization and highlights the key patterns and trends in news discourse, but it does not thoroughly examine audience reception to news articles on this topic (Seale 2003). Studies of audience reception are notoriously onerous to conduct and often involve research participants reacting to news articles in fabricated settings that bear little resemblance to the ways that people engage with news in the everyday of the digital news era. However, empirical attention to how news articles about

HIV criminalization resonate with readers may have offered meaningful insights into the social life of news on this topic.

A final limitation that relates to scope concerns the range of media discourses I consider in this book. I focus my analytic attention on crime genre news accounts of HIV criminalization in this project because these are the types of news stories that HIV advocates are seriously concerned about. In email correspondence among HIV activists I work with and within meetings of HIV organizations I am a part of, participants express alarm when someone's mugshot appears in a major daily news publication and when articles are produced as short, decontextualized crime stories. This means that this book does not address other types of news discourse about HIV criminalization (editorials, long-form opinion pieces, interviews with and features of HIV advocates, expert commentaries on legal decisions, etc.) or other forms of media representation of HIV criminalization (activist zines, publications of AIDS service organizations, popular depictions of this issue in television shows, etc.) in as much detail. This breadth of media on HIV criminalization is important and warrants further sociological analysis.

With an awareness of this book's limitations in mind, I hope that this work can contribute in useful ways to ongoing discussions that researchers and activists are having about what is to come for institutional ethnography, the ongoing struggle to end HIV criminalization, and the continuing production and circulation of harmful, stigmatizing health messages. To close, I reflect on what this book might add to dialogues in these areas.

What's Next for Institutional Ethnography? And What Can an IE Tell Us about the Ongoing Struggle to End HIV Criminalization?

At the outset of this book, I listed questions that typify the kinds of issues institutional ethnographers seem to be grappling with in the present moment. Questions along the lines of: What makes IE a distinct approach to sociology? What is IE's radical critique of sociology? What is IE's relationship to other sociologies? And how might we apply IE in ways that contribute to activist projects? It often seems that these questions derive from a rather anxious place. In my experience these questions are not typically posed as straightforward methodological questions. Rather, they are frequently couched in broader discussions about the stability and durability of the IE project overall and concerns about the extent to which IE will maintain secure footing and widespread recognition as an influential approach to social inquiry.

It may be that these questions are more pressing and perhaps feel more urgent since June 2022 when Dorothy Smith, the ground-breaking, feminist, Marxist sociologist who invented IE and taught the approach to generations of researchers and activists, died at the age of ninety-five. For decades, it was likely that one who studied IE had a profoundly unique type of relationship to the founder of their field. For reasons that have to do with the culture of celebrity intelligentsias or temporal and geographic divides, the founders of the fields we study are not typically thought of as accessible, approachable figures. For obvious reasons students of biopolitics are not going to happen upon and strike up a chat with Michel Foucault between sessions at the Canadian Congress of the Humanities and Social Sciences. However, for generations of IE students, especially those studying in Canada, it was not unusual to run into Dorothy in the hallways at conferences or to sit near her while attending presentations at IE sessions. She was an astonishingly generous mentor to the field of IE. Well into her nineties she wrote and presented papers at conferences, asked careful questions, and offered deeply thoughtful, bighearted feedback on paper presentations and draft manuscripts people shared with her. She somehow balanced an unwavering commitment to the core tenets of IE, while at the same time modelling the humility to acknowledge, and even encourage us to push those boundaries.

Her absence has rendered a tremendous void in the IE community, and I think it has left many of us wondering what's next for the project she started. The process of applying IE to produce knowledge for the movement to end HIV criminalization has shaped my understanding of the activist potential of IE and ways that we might articulate the unique utility of its approach to studying the social.

Institutional ethnography is often posited to pose a radical critique of mainstream sociology. At the same time, one would be right to point out that the field of sociology has undergone tremendous changes since IE emerged and to question if IE is still a radical alternative to "mainstream sociology," or if the approach has lost its contemporary relevance.[1] I think it is crucial to not lose sight of or take for granted the radial alternative that IE continues to offer to other sociologies. Here I have in mind the "ontological shift" that George Smith wrote about,

---

1 This question was among those posed during a recent panel I was part of at XX ISA World Congress of Sociology (29 June 2023) organized by Lauren Eastwood and Liza McCoy. My reflections in this chapter are derived from my responses to questions from the panel.

the materialist, feminist insistence on starting inquiry in the material reality of people's lives and treating people as expert knowers of their social worlds. While IE has grown into a broader collective project over the last thirty years and now spans global boarders and disciplinary boundaries, its transformative potential continues to lie in the notion that sociological relevance can be found in one's everyday communities and among the daily lives and struggles of activist collectives one works with.

My understanding of the activist potential of an IE project is rooted primarily in George Smith's seminal essay "Political Activist as Ethnographer." His work provides a model for how an institutional ethnographer can (1) base their research in the everyday lives of individuals, (2) develop an understanding of how these everyday lives are socially organized, and then (3) use research findings to inform actual interventions into the workings of a ruling regime. My study of mainstream news media discourse about HIV criminalization is premised on these three principles from Smith's essay. First, the project started in the everyday, local experiences of activists who were concerned with this genre of news reporting and looking to change how the issue was written about in the press. The sociological relevancy of this project was not determined by a review of sociological literature on news media discourse, rather it was the alarm and frustration of people mobilizing against HIV criminalization that guided the research. Second, the project was not a study of people as objects of research, and instead concentrated on the social organization of ruling relations. That is, the project was about showing how a common genre of news story about HIV criminalization is accomplished through everyday work practices that are coordinated across time and space.

The third, and perhaps most significant, principle from George Smith's essay is the attention he devotes to illustrating how IE can go to work for community activists. As he explains, "starting from the local, particular settings in the everyday world, the work of the activist ethnographer is to extend his or her member's knowledge to grasp how a ruling regime works with a view to transforming it" (1990, 629, 631). For IE to remain a meaningful radical alternative to other sociologies, we must preserve and foreground this feature of its approach to studying the social. That is, we ought to underline that IE is about ethnographically reporting "how things work" *and* about making social change by producing knowledge for social movements.

The knowledge that this IE produced about the social organization of the mainstream press can help to inform activist interventions into news coverage of HIV criminal non-disclosure cases. For example, the preceding chapters offer empirical evidence that:

1 In order to meaningfully alter the way that HIV is reported on in the mainstream press, the voices of people living with HIV must be at the forefront of advocacy interventions. When talking to reporters during fieldwork for this project, they expressed time and time again that in order to produce news stories that counter crime genre reports with longer-form, nuanced descriptions of criminal legal regulation of HIV disclosure, they require personal narratives that help readers "put a face" to this issue. HIV advocacy organizations would be well served to continue offering media training programs to support people living with HIV who want to enter into media discourse. HIV organizations should also ensure that HIV advocates not only have opportunities to have their voices included as part of news texts that reporters write but are also supported in the work of authoring their own media articles in the form of opinion editorials and letters to the editor. These types of media interventions can help ensure that people living with HIV are central to driving and defining media discourse.

2 HIV advocates looking to intervene in media discourse on HIV criminalization should be alert for opportunities to work within mainstream media. This means working within the structures of convergence journalism with an understanding that reporters' writing for digital news is often an exercise in copy and pasting other texts into news stories. Interventions that take on this approach may concentrate on producing texts (such as factsheets) that can compete with those published by criminal justice authorities that are often most readily available to reporters. This makes it more likely for advocates' voices to be included in news texts that hurried reporters produce.

3 Advocates should balance efforts to work within the confines of news media with projects that work against the mainstream press by broadcasting their messaging through independent publishing, zines, social media campaigns, in-person community forums, and other outlets. Representatives of a number of HIV organizations I interviewed described that they have (for good reason) grown so frustrated with the long lineage of racist, stigmatizing discourses in the news that they've largely jettisoned the mainstream press altogether and concentrate on securing funding to produce their own media content. These media products can be highly successful and circulate widely.

4   Given the ongoing overrepresentation of African, Caribbean, and Black defendants in newspaper coverage of HIV criminal non-disclosure cases, organizations that represent these communities have an important and unique role to play in developing and mobilizing forms of counter-discourse. Producing a consistent and coherent discourse to oppose HIV criminalization is challenging, resource-intensive work. And so, the efforts of collectives that represent African, Caribbean, and Black communities deserve and require collective, widespread support.

At the outset of this IE, I hoped that the project would uncover insights about news media discourse, such as the points above, that could go to work for activists. It has been encouraging to be part of community-based meetings and projects where activists draw on these kinds of findings as they strategize ways to respond when problematic coverage of an HIV criminal non-disclosure case circulates online or work to mobilize counter-discourses.[2]

However, at the time I began studying news discourse about HIV criminalization, I could not have foreseen the ways that researching and writing this book would coincide with a significant shift in Canadian policymakers' attitudes on this issue. While I carried out this project, governments started to acknowledge the broad harms associated with HIV criminalization that activists had been voicing for decades and even commenced a nationwide consultation to examine changes to the criminal code. These developments offered new avenues to mobilize knowledge from this project within activist movements to end HIV criminalization. Whereas early activist media work I was part of focused exclusively on how to respond to and shape news coverage of HIV criminal non-disclosure cases in particular, more recent work has been about how to engage with media as part of the broad effort to promote law reform on HIV criminalization. This kind of work commonly centres on questions regarding when, how, and if advocates should accept interview requests, respond to problematic news articles that are published, craft op-ed articles, contact journalists, and train activists to work as spokespeople during a monumental and delicate stage of the advocacy process.

The ways that activists drew on knowledge from this IE changed and expanded as the political context they encountered shifted.

---

2 See, for example, the HIV Legal Network's (2020) guide to media reporting on HIV and the criminal law.

During this time, the knowledge from the project that was valuable to activists did not only have to do with showing social organization, but instead, was about insights I gathered while interfacing with the ruling regime of news media. My time conducting institutional ethnographic fieldwork helped me learn about who the key reporters on this issue are, which reporters and publications would be most receptive to activists' messages, how particular aspects of activists' work might play amid certain news cycles, and how to frame complex legal arguments for mass audiences. My fieldwork also occasioned opportunities to communicate with reporters directly and to express the damaging effects of the standard genre of news writing about HIV criminalization. In one particularly promising instance, members of the CCRHC media working group and I emailed a reporter who had written a rather stigmatizing news story about HIV criminalization in which we included findings from this project and the HIV Legal Network's guide to media reporting on HIV and the criminal law. We were pleased when we received a response that outlined changes the news organization would be making to avoid producing this kind of coverage in the future

Other institutional ethnographers have recognized how the knowledge gained from interfacing with ruling regimes while doing an IE can go to work for activists. In his seminal essay, George Smith highlights that an often-overlooked aspect of IE's activist potential is that the practice of focusing analysis on ruling regimes often requires a fair amount of face-to-face occasions to collect data and efforts to recover knowledge from members who work within a regime. Similarly, in Viviane Namaste's (2006, 165) study of the process of name and sex changes for transgender people in Quebec she describes, "the research process itself involved a certain amount of interface between transsexuals and the government. Interviews with bureaucrats sent a clear message that their polices, as well as the changing interpretations of their policies, were under close scrutiny both by individual transsexuals as well as health researchers."

The activist utility of interfacing with ruling regimes is not often included in methodological descriptions of IE or in reports of social organization. However, I would suggest that these kinds of contributions that extend beyond only showing social organization must be central to how we articulate the scope and potential of IE. It is one of the ways that the radical alternative that IE offers to mainstream sociology can be illuminated. This is especially important in light of the contemporary challenges IE confronts in the Canadian context. Currently, IE does not have a stronghold in Canadian sociology. IE is mostly taught in professionalized spaces (nursing, education, social work). This makes sense given the tremendous influence that institutional ethnographies have had in these areas. At the same time, underlining the unique ways that IE produces knowledge that can go to work for activists can help spark dialogues between IE and other sociologies committed to social change (including settler colonial studies, critical race studies, gender studies, and others) and encourage dialogues about how IE can be taken up and applied to the most pressing and urgent social justice issues against which social movements struggle today.

The Continuing Production and Circulation of Harmful, Stigmatizing Health Messages

As we reflect on what IE can offer to social movements broadly, and the movement to end HIV criminalization in particular, it is worth considering how we might mobilize findings from this project to emerging social justice issues that lie at the intersection of public health, law, and mass media. For one, we would do well to keep in mind that those who are working to ensure that news content about public health issues is informed by social justice and human rights principles do so at a time when the relationship between public health information, the mainstream press, and the circulation of news online is highly fraught. It has been remarkable to witness (and try to intervene in) how the social relations of online news and public health have become knotted together over the course of this project. I began fieldwork for this project just weeks after "fake news" was named as the word of the year in 2017, and widespread trust in the mainstream news seemed to be at an all-time low. The first drafts of writing that emerged from that fieldwork were completed in March 2020 as many parts of our lives were rescheduled, cancelled, and moved online.

In the weeks that followed the early days of COVID-19, many of us started to know and understand how to live our daily lives during the pandemic by way of news reports that tracked how the virus was moving across the globe and into our communities and helped to make sense of public health guidance. News media articles likely guided many of our first experiences of masking, distancing, testing, and yes, perhaps even scrubbing our groceries as they entered our homes. At the same time, public health officials also cautioned that misinformation and "fake news" lurk within accounts of COVID-19 that circulate online and warned of a growing "infodemic" that accompanied the rapidly evolving global public health emergency. As Tedros Adhanom Ghebreyesus, director-general of the World Health Organization (WHO) explained: "We're not just fighting an epidemic; we're fighting an infodemic." Public health organizations took to employing virologic imagery to liken the threat of an infodemic to that of the pandemic itself. For example, WHO defined the "infodemic" as "an overabundance of information and the rapid spread of misleading or fabricated news … like the virus, it is highly contagious and grows exponentially. It also complicates COVID-19 pandemic response efforts." Here, we can once again recognize how the relations of commercialized convergence journalism are not aligned with public health. While a lot of news about COVID-19 helped to clarify and inform thoughtful, evidence-based responses to the pandemic, other types of news media have produced confusing, sensational, and inaccurate narratives about the virus that muddled efforts to curb its spread.

Almost two years into a global pandemic, I'm writing the conclusion to this book from my home in Montreal, where just a few hours down the road, a "freedom convoy" led by hate groups and truckers has ensnarled Ottawa. Demonstrators are against vaccine mandates and are demanding "the federal government end all mandates, as they view that like other pandemic restrictions, they infringe on our freedoms." The images of the siege are disheartening. Along with reports of constantly blaring truck horns and late-night fireworks, Ottawa residents have recounted personal threats, harassment, intimidation, hateful vitriol, and signage from "protestors." In the early days of the convoy, a friend who lives in Ottawa posted photos he took of the blockade on social media. An image of the back of a red truck cab stood out to me. The cab is lit by yellow and red running lights and two large gas canisters are affixed to the truck bed. Above the gas canisters, scrawled in the grime that has built up on the cab is a message that reads: "MEDIA IS THE VIRUS."

This IE might offer lessons about making sense of how it possibly comes to be that WHO leaders and "freedom convoy" "demonstrators" land on similar virologic metaphors to express frustrations about how media circulates information (or fails to do so) about a pandemic. For one, it underlines the importance of buttressing studies of news content, that are useful for alerting us to "infodemics," with studies of social organization that help illustrate how these stories are produced and circulate. Much like the case of HIV criminalization, an institutional ethnographer would want to think and investigate across a wide complex of institutional sites. These might include social media platforms, digital audience analytic programs that are employed in newsrooms, newsrooms themselves, and public health organizations, to name a few. My hope is that this book in some way contributes to a long lineage of IE research that offers possibilities for extending understandings of how we can intervene in complicated, weighty situations such as this.

Research Methods

This book is based in sociological institutional ethnographic field research that involved watching what happened, listening to what people said, asking questions about what people do, and collecting data over an extended period of time in an effort to learn about how news stories about HIV criminalization are produced (Hammersley and Atkinson 1995). The project received research ethics approval from York University. The fieldwork that I conducted between 2015 and 2018 involved extensive reading of news articles about HIV criminalization, participating in community-based HIV advocacy groups' meetings and conferences, and thirty-five interviews with people who shape news stories. I interviewed twenty journalists, fourteen HIV advocates, and one police communications representative. It is important to note that some of the participants occupy multiple roles; for example, I spoke with activists who produced news content in the form of opinion-editorial articles. Of the thirty-five interviews that I conducted, segments of thirty are included in this book. I selected these thirty accounts because they most clearly reflected the trends that I recognized across the corpus of interview transcripts and made visible how work that was taking place in one social location was hooked up to work that others were doing in other social sites.

I recruited interview participants in an assortment of ways. Prior to beginning fieldwork, I did not have experience in the social world of news production, so it was challenging to enlist journalists to speak with. I sent cold emails to reporters who had written on the issue of HIV criminalization in the past five years and those who authored articles that were published during my fieldwork. This process enabled me to recruit twelve reporters to the study. It was common for interview participants to recommend other journalists for me to interview, and this helped to broaden the range of news reporters I spoke with. I also posted an open call on social media for individuals who work in news media available to participate in an interview.

Most of the reporters I interviewed work for what can broadly be understood as "mainstream" news organizations. There are various ways that scholars define and theorize "mainstream" news. For instance, some scholars differentiate mainstream news from alternative news in terms of the size of the audience (Turow 1997). These scholars view mainstream media outlets as those that broadcast to the largest possible share of the public audience, whereas alternative media narrowcast to specific small-scale niche audiences (Tsfati and Peri 2006, 168). Other scholars distinguish mainstream news from alternative news with reference to ownership. In this sense, mainstream media are owned by large corporations, whereas alternative media are smaller-scale news productions with less funding (Shoemaker 2001). Most scholars who study mainstream media understand the mainstream/ alternative media dichotomy to reflect the distance between power centres in society. Whereas mainstream media are viewed as embedded in power, alternative media channels reflect views that are seldom heard on mainstream channels (Atton 2002; Downing 2001; Shoemaker 2001). While it is challenging to mark clear and consistent distinctions between mainstream and alternative news, of the twenty reporters I interviewed, fourteen work for organizations that generally fit the characteristics of mainstream news outlined here. That is, they work for organizations that produce and broadcast news content for mass audiences, are owned and operated by large corporations (either government or privately owned), and communicate news stories that reflect power relations in society.

HIV criminalization has been thoughtfully covered in alternative presses, zines, and activist publications (Black and Whitbread 2018; How to Have Sex in a Police State: One Approach, n.d.; Keogh 2017; McClelland 2019b; Ritchie 2017). This issue has also been attentively addressed in long-form, mainstream news publications that diverge from quick, crime genre stories. However, this book focuses mostly on the work of reporters who broadcast crime genre stories for two reasons: first, because these are the stories about which activists have expressed the most consistent concern and alarm, and second, because most stories about HIV criminalization are written as crime stories (Mykhalovskiy et al. 2016, 33). Thus, most accounts of newswork included in this book are descriptions of concise and fast writing for digital news. This also means that this project offers fewer insights into the particularities of producing longer-form journalism or alternative news content.

Recruiting HIV advocates to interview was a much more straight-forward process than accessing reporters. I enlisted participants by reviewing news articles about HIV criminalization and contacting those who appeared in news stories as spokespeople. I knew many of these individuals through my extended network of people who work as HIV activists, community organizers, legal experts, lawyers, and researchers in the field of HIV. Ultimately, cold emails, the snowballing method, and the social media call yielded an about even distribution of participants.

All interviews were recorded and transcribed in full. Interviews were typically forty-five minutes to an hour in length – the shortest interview was twenty minutes, and the longest was an hour and fifteen minutes. Some journalists kept in touch and shared with me subsequent news articles that they published. I continue to work alongside many of the HIV advocates I interviewed on community-based working groups and collectives.

Interviewees are referred to in this book by pseudonyms.[1] To protect the anonymity of research participants who work in the field of journalism, I have altered the names of news organizations, publications, headlines, and details of news stories that they named during interviews. Similarly, I have also changed the names of community-based HIV advocacy organizations that activists spoke about during our discussions. HIV advocates and researchers have repeatedly called on journalists to avoid publishing the names of people who face criminal charges for not disclosing their HIV-positive status, because this press coverage can cause a litany of long-term harms. In this book, I have sought to protect the anonymity of those who have faced charges by using pseudonyms and altering details of criminal cases, such as the year in which criminal charges happened and the location in which they occurred.

The interviews did not follow a structured list of questions, except for one interview in which an individual participated on the condition that they receive a list of questions ahead of the interview and that our conversation not stray from that list. My approach to interviewing was informed by interview methods for institutional ethnographic research. Institutional ethnographic interviews are not standardized and are perhaps best described as "talking with people" as part of a "fully reflexive

---

1 Research participants from the Canadian HIV/AIDS Legal Network agreed to waive anonymity. Because of the specificity of their work, it would have been challenging to ensure their anonymity.

process in which both the participant and the interviewer construct knowledge together" (DeVault and McCoy 2004, 24). The most distinctive feature of interviews in institutional ethnographic research is that they focus on the work that people do. I related to interviews as a way to learn about what people's everyday activities consist of, how they know how to carry out those activities, and how that work is hooked up to broader ruling relations. This meant starting interviews by asking journalists to broadly describe a "typical workday" or prompting an HIV advocate to "take me through how you and your organization crafted a response to this news report about HIV criminalization." Because I sought detailed accounts of respondents' work practices and wanted to learn about how their work is hooked up to work that happens elsewhere, I often interjected to ask questions such as "How did you know to complete that step of your work process?"; "What do you mean by that?"; "Can you share examples of what that looks like?" This was important for gaining an understanding of what particular people's actual work consists of and identifying how it connects to work done by other people in other social settings.

I used NVivo software to organize interview transcripts and field notes but did not use discrete coding categories to analyse data. Instead, I read interview transcripts for social organization. Reading for how speakers' accounts are socially organized means being attentive to the form of activity that is represented in one's talk and to the relations that make that activity possible (Mykhalovskiy and McCoy 2002, 29). This involves posing questions that direct analytic attention to how people's activities interface with broad social relations that shape them. For example, in my analysis I asked how it is that reporters' work to decide that an item is newsworthy comes to involve the work of reading police documents and "wondered about the social and institutional relations that made such work possible and that are entered into by the speaker in his or her doing of that work" (30).

References

ACT. n.d. *History of ACT: A Summary of ACT's History Since Its Founding in 1983*. Accessed 25 April 2022. https://www.actoronto.org/about-act/our -history/.

Adam, Barry D.. Patrice Corriveau, Richard Elliott, Jason Globerman, Ken English, and Sean Rourke. 2015. "HIV Disclosure as Practice and Public Policy." *Critical Public Health* 25, no. 4 (August): 386–97. https://doi.org /10.1080/09581596.2014.980395.

– 2016. "HIV Positive People's Perspectives on Canadian Criminal Law and Non-Disclosure." *Canadian Journal of Law & Society* 31, no. 1 (April): 1–23. https://doi.org/10.1017/cls.2016.3.

Adam, Barry D , Richard Elliott, Patrice Corriveau, and Ken English. 2014. "Impacts of Criminalization on the Everyday Lives of People Living with HIV in Canada." *Sexuality Research and Social Policy* 11, no. 1 (March): 39–49. https://doi.org/10.1007/s13178-013-0131-8.

African and Caribbean Council on HIV/AIDS in Ontario. 2013. *Our Voices: HIV, Race, and the Criminal Law*. Toronto: African and Caribbean Council on HIV/AIDS in Ontario.

AIDS Activist History Project. n.d. *AIDS ACTION NOW!* Accessed 25 April 2022. https://aidsactivisthistory.ca/features/george-w-smith/aids-action -now/.

Alang, Sirry, Donna McAlpine, Ellen McCreedy, and Rachel Hardeman. 2017. "Police Brutality and Black Health: Setting the Agenda for Public Health Scholars." *American Journal of Public Health* 107, no. 5 (May): 662–5. https:// doi.org/10.2105/AJPH.2017.303691.

Albert, Edward. 1986. "Acquired Immune Deficiency Syndrome: The Victim and the Press." *Studies in Communication* 3: 135–58.

Allain, Carol Ann. 1988. "AIDS Update What Black Women Need to Know about AIDS " *Our Lives: Canada's First Black Women's Newspaper* (Spring): 5.

Almiron, Nuria. 2010. *Journalism in Crisis: Corporate Media and Financialization*. New York: Hampton Press.

Altheide, David L. 2003. "Mass Media, Crime, and the Discourse of Fear." *Hedgehog Review* 5, no. 3 (Fall): 9–25.

Ananny, Mike, and Megan Finn. 2020. "Anticipatory News Infrastructures: Seeing Journalism's Expectations of Future Publics Inits Sociotechnical Systems." *New Media and Society* 22, no. 9 (September): 1600–18. https://doi.org/10.1177/1461444820914873.

Anderson, C.W. 2013. "Towards a Sociology of Computational and Algorithmic Journalism." *New Media and Society* 15, no. 7 (November): 1005–21. https://doi.org/10.1177/1461444812465137.

Atton, Chris. 2002. *Alternative Media*. London: Sage. https://doi.org/10.4135/9781446220153.

Bains, Camille. 2019. "Advocates Call on Provinces to Develop Consistent Policies on Limiting HIV Prosecutions." *Globe and Mail*, 4 February. https://www.theglobeandmail.com/canada/article-advocates-call-on-provinces-to-develop-consistent-policies-on-limiting/.

Baker, Andrea J. 1986. "The Portrayal of AIDS in the Media: An Analysis of Articles in the New York Times." In *Social Dimension of AIDS: Method and Theory*, edited by Douglas A. Feldman and Thomas A. Johnson, 179–94. New York: Praeger.

Bakker, Piet. 2012. "Aggregation, Content Farms, and Huffinization." *Journalism Practice* 6, nos. 5–6 (October): 627–37. https://doi.org/10.1080/17512786.2012.667266.

Barnett, Steven. 2009. *Journalism, Democracy, and the Public Interest: Rethinking Media Pluralism for the Digital Age*. Oxford: Reuters Institute for the Study of Journalism.

Barré-Sinoussi, François, Salim S. Abdool Karim, Jan Albert, Linda-Gail Bekker, Chris Beyrer, Pedro Cahn, Alexandra Calmy, Beatriz Grinsztejn, Andrew Grulich, Adeeba Kamarulzaman, et al. 2018. "Expert Consensus Statement on the Science of HIV in the Context of Criminal Law." *Journal of the International AIDS Society* 21, no. 7 (July): e25161. https://doi.org/10.1002/jia2.25161.

Batsell, Jake. 2015. *Engaged Journalism: Connecting with Digitally Empowered News Audiences*. New York: Columbia University Press.

Bayer, Ronald. 1991. Review of Covering the Plague: AIDS and the American Media, by James Kinsella. *AIDS Education and Prevention* 3, no. 1: 74–86.

Beale, Sara Sun. 2006. "The News Media's Influence on Criminal Justice Policy: How Market-Driven News Promotes Punitiveness." *William and Mary Law Review* 48, no. 2: 397–481.

Beck, Ulrich. 1992. *The Risk Society*. London: Sage.

Beeston, Laura. 2017. "Advocates Hope for Change in HIV Non-Disclosure Law After Ottawa Meeting with Provinces." *Toronto Star*, 5 March 2017. https://www.thestar.com/news/gta/advocates-hope-for-change-in-hiv -non-disclosure-law-after-ottawa-meeting-with-provinces/article_0506560d -bcf6-5444-9aa9-d7840b14f5c7.html.

Beger, Randall R. 2002. "Expansion of Police Power in Public Schools and the Vanishing Rights of Students." *Social Justice* 29, nos. 1–2: 119–30.

Bell, Emily. 2016. "Facebook Is Eating the World." *Columbia Journalism Review*, 7 March 2016. https://www.cjr.org/analysis/facebook_and_media.php.

Bell, Niko. 2017. "Should Toronto Police Publish Names of People Charged with Not Disclosing Their HIV Status?" *Xtra*, 13 July 2017. https://www .dailyxtra.com/should-toronto-police-publish-names-of-people-charged -with-not-disclosing-their-hiv-status-76150.

Benbunan-Fich, Raquel, and Eliezer M. Fich. 2004. "Effects of Web Traffic Announcements on Firm Value." *International Journal of Electronic Commerce* 8, no. 4 (October): 161–31. https://doi.org/10.1080/10864415.2004 .11044312.

Bernard, Edwin J., Alison Symington, and Sylvie Beaumont. 2022. "Punishing Vulnerability Through HIV Criminalization." *American Journal of Public Health* 112, no. S4 (June): S395–7. https://doi.org/10.2105/AJPH.2022.306713.

Bilton, Ricardo. 2015. "The Golden Age of Journalism – For Millennial Reporters, That Is." *Digiday*, 4 June 2015. https://digiday.com/media /golden-age-journalism-millennial-reporters/.

Bird, S. Elizabeth, and Robert W. Dardenne. 2009. "Rethinking News and Myth as Storytelling." In *Handbook of Journalism Studies*, edited by Karin Wahl-Jorgensen and Thomas Hanitzsch, 205–17. New York: Routledge.

Black, Anthea, and Jessica Whitbread. 2018. "Criminalization-Medicalization." *The HIV Howler*, no. 1

Blatchford, Christie. 2008. "HIV-Positive Man Was 'Actively Involved' Patient Concerned with His Well-Being, Specialist Testifies." *Globe and Mail*, 22 October, A7.

Boesman, Jan, and Irene Costera Meijer. 2018. "Nothing But the Facts? Exploring the Discursive Space for Storytelling and Truth-Seeking in Journalism." *Journalism Practice* 12, no. 8 (September): 997–1007. https:// doi.org/10.1080/17512786.2018.1493947.

Bogosavljevic, Katarina, and Jennifer M. Kilty. 2017. "Justice Isn't Blind on HIV Non-Disclosure." *Winnipeg Free Press*, 1 December, A

Boyd, Rhea W. 2018. "Police Violence and the Built Harm of Structural Racism." *Lancet* 392, no. 10144 (28 July): 258–9. https://doi.org/10.1016 /S0140-6736(18)31374-6.

Braun, Joshua A. 2015. *This ProgramIs Brought to You by …: Distributing Television News Online*. New Haven, CT: Yale University Press. https://doi.org/10.12987/yale/9780300197501.001.0001.

Breed, Warren. 1955. "Social Control in the Newsroom: A Functional Analysis." *Social Forces* 33, no. 4 (May): 326–35. https://doi.org/10.2307/2573002.

Brock, Deborah, Amanda Glasbeek, and Carmela Murdocca, eds. 2014. *Criminalization, Representation, Regulation: Thinking Differently about Crime*. Toronto: University of Toronto Press.

Brock, George. 2013. *Out of Print: Newspapers, Journalism and the Business of News in the Digital Age*. London: Kogan Page.

Broersma, Marcel. 2010. "The Unbearable Limitations of Journalism." *The International Communication Gazette* 72, no. 1 (February): 21–33. https://doi.org/10.1177/1748048509350336.

Broersma, Marcel, and Chris Peters. 2012. "Rethinking Journalism: The Structural Transformation of a Public Good." In *Rethnking Journalism: Trust and Participation in a Transformed News Landscape*, edited by Chirs Peters and Marcel Broersma, 1–13. New York: Routledge.

Broersma, Marcel, and Jane B. Singer. 2021. "Caught between Innovation and Tradition: Young Journalists as Normative Change Agents in the Journalistic Field." Journalistic Practice 15, no. 6 (July): 821–38. https://doi.org/10.1080/17512786.2020.1824125.

Brown, George R. 2016. "The Blue Line on Thin Ice: Police Use of Force Modifications in the Era of Cameraphones and YouTube." *British Journal of Criminology* 56, no. 2 (March): 293–312. https://doi.org/10.1093/bjc/azv052.

Browne, Irene, Natalie Delia Deckard, and Cassaundra Rodriguez. 2016. "Different Game, Different Frame?: Black Counterdiscourses and Depictions of Immigration in Atlanta's African-American and Mainstream Press." *Sociological Quarterly* 57, no. 3 (August): 520–43. https://doi.org/10.1111/tsq.12146.

Burris, Scott, Leo Beletsky, Joseph A. Burleson, Patricia Case, and Zita Lazzarini. 2007. "Do Criminal Laws Influence HIV Risk Behavior? An Empirical Trial." *Arizona State Law Journal* 39, no. 2 (Summer): 467–517.

Camp, Jordan T., and Christina Heatherton. 2016. *Policing the Planet: Why the Policing Crisis Led to Black Lives Matter*. New York: Verso.

Campbell, Marie, and Frances Gregor. 2008. *Mapping Social Relations: A Primer in Doing Institutional Ethnography*. Toronto: University of Toronto Press.

Canadian HIV/AIDS Legal Network. 2014. *Criminal Law and HIV Non-Disclosure in Canada*. Toronto: Canadian HIV/AIDS Legal Network.

Canadian Institutes of Health Research. 2018. *CIHR HIV/AIDS Community-Based Research*. https://web.archive.org/web/20180620164300/https://cihr-irsc.gc.ca/e/25835.html.

The Canadian Press. 2017. "Would an HIV-Positive Woman Get Charged If She Was Raped? McMaster Prof Asks." *CBC News*, 16 January. https://www.cbc.ca/news/canada/hamilton/would-an-hiv-positive-woman-get-charged-if-she-was-raped-mcmaster-prof-asks-1.3937241.

Carney, Nikita. 2016. "All Lives Matter, But So Does Race: Black Lives Matter and the Evolving Role of Social Media." *Humanity and Society* 40, no. 2 (May): 180–200. https://doi.org/10.1177/0160597616643868.

Castells, Manuel. 2009a. *Communication Power*. New York: Oxford University Press.

Castells, Manuel. 2009b. *The Rise of the Network Society: The Information Age: Economy, Society, and Culture*. Malden, MA: Blackwell Publishing. https://doi.org/10.1002/9781444319514.

Chadha, Kalyani, and Rob Wells. 2016. "Journalistic Responses to Technological Innovation in Newsrooms." *Digital Journalism* 4, no. 8 (November): 1–16. https://doi.org/10.1080/21670811.2015.1123100.

Chan, Wendy, and Dorothy Chunn. 2014. *Racialization, Crime, and Criminal Justice in Canada*. Toronto: University of Toronto Press.

Chappell, Tauhid, and Mike Rispoli. 2020. "Defund the Crime Beat." *NiemanLab*. https://www.niemanlab.org/2020/12/defund-the-crime-beat/.

Cheng, Tony. 2021. "Social Media, Socialization, and Pursuing Legitimation of Police Violence." *Criminology* 59, no. 3 (August): 391–418. https://doi.org/10.1111/1745-9125.12277.

Chermak, Steven M. 1995. *Victims in the News: Crime and the American News Media*. Boulder, CO: Westview Press.

Chermak, Steven M., and Alexander Weiss. 2005. "Maintaining Legitimacy Using External Communication Strategies: An Analysis of Police-Media Relations." *Journal of Criminal Justice* 33, no. 5 (September–October): 501–12. https://doi.org/10.1016/j.jcrimjus.2005.06.001.

Christin, Angèle. 2020. *Metrics at Work: Journalism and the Contested Meaning of Algorithms*. Princeton NJ: Princeton University Press. https://doi.org/10.23943/princeton/9780691175232.001.0001.

Cooper, Hannah L.F., and Mindy Thompson Fullilove. 2020. *From Enforcers to Guardians: A Public Health Primer on Ending Police Violence*. Baltimore, MD: Johns Hopkins University Press.

Côté-Lussier, Carolyn. 2013. "Narratives of Legitimacy: Police Expansionism and the Contest Over Policing." *Policing and Society* 23, no. 2 (June): 183–203. https://doi.org/10.1080/10439463.2012.671820.

Coxon, Lisa. 2013. "What We Lose When Newspapers Give Up on Beat Reporting." *J Source: The Canadian Journalism Project*, 4 December. https://j-source.ca/article/what-we-lose-when-newspapers-give-up-on-beat-reporting/.

Craig, Geoffrey. 2010. "Dialogue and Dissemination in News Media Interviews." *Journalism* 11, no. 1 (November): 75–90. https://doi.org/10.1177/1464884909349582.

Davies, Nick. 2008. *Flat Earth News*. London: Chatto and Windus.

Deleuze, Gilles, and Claire Parnet. 1977. *Dialogues*. Paris: Flammarion.

Dépelteau, François. 2018. "Relational Thinking in Sociology: Relevance, Concurrence and Dissonance." In *The Palgrave Handbook of Relational Sociology*, edited by François Dépelteau, 3–34. Cham, Switzerland: Palgrave Macmillan. https://doi.org/10.1007/978-3-319-66005-9_1.

DeVault, Marjorie, and Liza McCoy. 2006. "Using Interviews to Investigate Ruling Relations." In *Institutional Ethnography in Practice*, edited by Dorothy Smith, 15–44. Lanham, MD: Rowman and Littlefield.

Dixon, Travis L. 2018. *A Dangerous Distortion of Our Families: Representations of Families, by Race, in News and Opinion Media – December 2017*. Oakland, CA: Family Story and Color of Strange. https://colorofchange.org/dangerousdistortion/.

Dodds, Catherine, Adam Bourne, and Matthew Weait. 2009. "Responses to Criminal Prosecutions for HIV Transmission among Gay Men with HIV in England and Wales." *Reproductive Health Matters* 17, no. 34 (November): 135–45. https://doi.org/10.1016/S0968-8080(09)34475-4.

Dodds, Catherine, and Peter Keogh. 2006. "Criminal Prosecutions for HIV Transmission: People Living with HIV Respond." *STD & AIDS* 17, no. 5 (May): 315–18. https://doi.org/10.1258/095646206776790114.

Dodds, Catherine, Matthew Weait, Adam Bourne, and Siri Egede. 2015. "Keeping Confidence: HIV and the Criminal Law from HIV Service Providers' Perspectives." *Critical Public Health* 25, no. 4 (August): 410–26. https://doi.org/10.1080/09581596.2015.1019835.

Downing, John D.H. 2001. *Radical Media*. Thousand Oaks, CA: Sage.

Doyle, Gillian. 2013. "Re-Invention and Survival: Newspapers in the Era of Digital Multiplatform Delivery." *Journal of Media Business Studies* 10, no. 4 (December): 1–20. https://doi.org/10.1080/16522354.2013.11073569.

Easton, Rob. 2016. "Canadian News Coverage of HIV Assaults Proven to Be Racist." *Canadaland*, 28 November. https://www.canadalandshow.com/canadian-news-coverage-hiv-assaults-proven-racist/.

Eichaelberger, Laura. 2007. "SARS and New York's Chinatown: The Politics of Risk and Blame During an Epidemic of Fear." *Social Science and Medicine* 65, no. 6 (September): 1284–95. https://doi.org/10.1016/j.socscimed.2007.04.022.

Emirbayer, Mustafa. 1997. "Manifesto for a Relational Sociology." *American Journal of Sociology* 103, no. 2 (September): 281–317. https://doi.org/10.1086/231209.

Emmanuel, Rachel. 2019. "Lawmakers Urge Ottawa to Amend Criminal Code Around HIV." *Globe and Mail*, 24 June. https://theglobeandmail.com/politics/article-lawmakers-urge-ottawa-to-amend-criminal-code-around-hiv/.

Entman, Robert M. 1992. "Blacks in the News: Television, Modern Racism, and Cultural Change." *Journal of Communication* 69, no. 2 (June): 341–61. https://doi.org/10.1177/107769909206900209.

– 1993. "Framing: Toward Clarification of a Fractured Paradigm." *Journal of Communication* 43, no. 4 (December): 51–8. https://doi.org/10.1111/j.1460-2466.1993.tb01304.x.

– 1994. "African Americans According to TV News." *Media Studies Journal* 8, no. 3 (Summer): 29–38.

– 2003. "Cascading Activation: Contesting the White House's Frame After 9/11." *Political Communication* 20, no. 4 (October): 415–32. https://doi.org/10.1080/10584600390244176.

Ericson, Richard V. 1988. "How Journalists Visualize Fact." *Annals of the American Academy of Political and Social Science* 560, no. 1 (November): 83–95. https://doi.org/10.1177/0002716298560001007.

– 1994. "The Division of Expert Knowledge in Policing and Security." *British Journal of Sociology* 45, no. 2 (June): 149–75. https://doi.org/10.2307/591490.

Ericson, Richard V., Patricia M. Baranek, and Janet B.L. Chan. 1989. *Negotiating Control: A Study of News Sources*. Toronto: University of Toronto Press.

– 1991. *Representing Order: Crime, Law, and Justice in the News Media*. Toronto: University of Toronto Press.

Feltwell, Tom, John Vines, Karen Salt, Mark Blythe, Ben Kirman, Julie Barnett, Phillip Brooker, and Shaun Lawson. 2017. "Counter-Discourse Activism on Social Media: The Case of Challenging 'Poverty Porn' Television." *Computer Supported Cooperative Work* 26, no. 3 (June): 345–85. https://doi.org/10.1007/s10606-017-9275-z.

Fenlon, Brodie. 2021. "Canadian Trust in Journalism Is Wavering. Here's What CBC News Is Doing about It." *CBC News*, 4 March. https://www.cbc.ca/news/editorsblog/editor-blog-trust-1.5936535.

Flavin, Jeanne. 2000. "(Mis)Representing Risk: Headline Accounts of HIV-Related Assaults." *American Journal of Criminal Justice* 25, no. 1 (September): 119–36.

Fleming, Paul J., William D. Lopez, Maren Spolum, Riana Elyse Anderson, Angela G. Reyes, and Amy J. Schulz. 2021. "Policing Is a Public Health Issue: The Important Role of Health Educators." *Health Education &Behavior* 48, no. 5 (October): 553–8. https://doi.org/10.1177/10901981211001010.

Foucault, Michel. 1970. *The Archaeology of Knowledge*. New York: Pantheon.

Fraser, Nancy. 1990. "Rethinking the Public Sphere: A Contribution to the Critique of Actually Existing Democracy." *Social Text*, nos. 25/26: 56–80. https://doi.org/10.2307/466240.

French, Martin. 2015. "Counselling Anomie: Clashing Govermentalities of HIV Criminalization and Prevention." *Critical Public Health* 25, no. 4 (August): 427–40.

Fry, Hedy. 2017. *Disruption: Change and Churning in Canada's Media Landscape – Report of the Standing Committee on Canadian Heritage*. Ottawa: House of Commons. https://www.ourcommons.ca/documentviewer/en/42-1/CHPC/report-6/page-ToC.

Fuller, Jack. 2010. *What Is Happening to News: The Information Explosion and the Crisis in News*. Chicago: University of Chicago Press.

Gallagher, Ryan J., Andrew J. Reagan, Christopher M. Danforth, and Peter Sheridan Dodds. 2018. "Divergent Discourse Between Protests and Counter-Protests: #BlackLivesMatter and #AllLivesMatter." *PLoS ONE* 13, no. 4 (18 April): e0195644. https://doi.org/10.1371/journal.pone.0195644.

Gallant, Jacques. 2019. "Federal Committee Urges Changes to Curb HIV-Related Criminal Prosecutions." *Toronto Star*, 17 June. https://www.thestar.com/news/gta/federal-committee-urges-changes-to-curb-hiv-related-criminal-prosecutions/article_d4b07e2e-53d1-59c2-a1e2-5c696a10af71.html.

Galletly, Carol L., and Julia Dickson-Gomez. 2009. "HIV Seropositive Status Disclosure to Prospective Sex Partners and Criminal Laws That Require It: Perspectives of Persons Living with HIV." *STD & AIDS* 20, no. 9 (September): 613–18. https://doi.org/10.1258/ijsa.2008.008417.

Gans, Herbert J. 1979. *Deciding What's News: A Study of CBS Evening News, NBC Nightly News, Newsweek, and Time*. Medill School of Journalism. Evanston, IL: Northwestern University Press.

Garcia, Jennifer Jee-Lyn, and Mienah Zulfacar Sharif. 2015. "Black Lives Matter: A Commentary on Racism and Public Health." *American Journal of Public Health* 105, no. 8 (August): e27–e30. https://doi.org/10.2105/AJPH.2015.302706.

Giddens, Anthony. 1990. *The Consequences of Modernity*. Cambridge, UK: Polity.

– 1991. *Modernity and Self-Identity: Self and Society in the Late Modern Age*. Stanford: Stanford University Press.

Gilbert, Keon L., and Rashawn Ray. 2016. "Why Police Kill Black Males with Impunity: Applying Public Health Critical Race Praxis (PHCRP) to Address the Determinants of Policing Behaviors and 'Justifiable' Homicides in the USA." *Journal of Urban Health* 93, no. S1 (April): 122–40. https://doi.org/10.1007/s11524-015-0005-x.

Gillett, James. 2003. "Media Activism and Internet Use by People with HIV/AIDS." *Sociology of Health & Illness* 25, no. 6 (September): 608–24. https://doi.org/10.1111/1467-9566.00361.

Gitlan, Todd. 1980. *The Whole World Is Watching: Mass Media in the Making and Unmaking of the New Left*. Berkely: University of California Press.

Goffman, Erving. 1963. *Stigma: Notes on the Management of a Spoiled Identity*. New York: Simon & Schuster.

Goh, Su-Ling. 2017. "New Report Suggests Racism in Canadian Newspaper Articles About HIV." *Global News*, 9 February. https://globalnews.ca/news/3238558/new-report-suggests-racism-in-canadian-newspaper-articles-about-hiv/.

Gover, Angela R., Shannon B. Harper, and Lynn Langton. 2020. "Anti-Asian Hate Crime During the COVID-19 Pandemic: Exploring the Reproduction of Inequality." *American Journal of Criminal Justice* 45, no. 4 (August): 647–67. https://doi.org/10.1007/s12103-020-09545-1.

Grabosky, Peter, and Paul Wilson. 1989. *Journalism and Justice: How Crime Is Reported*. Leichhardt, AUS: Pluto Press.

Gramlick, John. 2016. "Voters' Perceptions of Crime Continue to Conflict with Reality." *Pew Research Center*, 16 November. https://www.pewresearch.org/fact-tank/2016/11/16/voters-perceptions-of-crime-continue-to-conflict-with-reality/.

Greenberg, Joshua. 2000. "Opinion Discourse and Canadian Newspapers: The Case of the Chinese 'Boat People.'" *Canadian Journal of Communication* 25, no. 4 (April): 517–37. https://doi.org/10.22230/cjc.2000v25n4a1178.

Hall, Stuart, Chas Cricher, Tony Jefferson, John Clarke, and Brian Roberts. 1978. *Policing the Crisis: Mugging, the State, and Law and Order*. London: Macmillan.

Hammersley, Martyn, and Paul Atkinson. 1995. "What Is Ethnography?" In *Ethnography: Principles in Practice*, 1–22. London: Routledge.

Hanusch, Folker, and C. Edson Tandoc, Jr. 2019. "Comments, Analytics, and Social Media: The Impact of Audience Feedback on Journalists' Market Orientation." *Journalism* 20, no. 6 (June): 695–713. https://doi.org/10.1177/1464884917720305.

Hastings, Colin. 2019. "The Social Relations of Disclosure: Critical Reflections on the Community-Based Response to HIV Criminalization." In *Thinking Differently About HIV/AIDS: Contributions from Critical Social Science*, edited by Eric Mykhalovskiy and Viviane Namaste, 278–302. Vancouver: UBC Press. https://doi.org/10.59962/9780774860727-011.

Hastings, Colin, Cécile Kazatchkine, and Eric Mykhalovskiy. 2017. *HIV Criminalization in Canada: Key Trends and Patterns*. Toronto: Canadian HIV/AIDS Legal Network.

Hastings, Colin, Notisha Massaquoi, Richard Elliott, and Eric Mykhalovskiy. 2022. *HIV Criminization in Canada: Key Trends and Patterns (1989–2020)*. Toronto: HIV Legal Network.

Hastings, Colin, and Eric Mykhalovskiy. 2023. "Reflections on Social Relations and the Single Institution Tendency in Institutional Ethnography." In *Critical Commentary on Institutional Ethnography: IE Scholars Speak to Its Promise*, edited by Paul C. Luken and Suzanne Vaughan, 69–90. Cham, Switzerland: Palgrave Macmillan. https://doi.org/10.1007/978-3-031-33402-3_5.

Hastings, Colin, Eric Mykhalovskiy, Chris Sanders, and Laura Bisaillon. 2020. "Disrupting a Canadian Prairie Fantasy and Constructing Racial Otherness: An Analysis of News Media Coverage of Trevis Smith's Criminal HIV Non-Disclosure Case." *Canadian Journal of Sociology* 45, no. 1 (March): 1–22. https://doi.org/10.29173/cjs29472.

Henry, Frances, and Carol Tator. 2002. *Discourse of Domination: Racial Bias in the Canadian English-Language Press*. Toronto: University of Toronto Press. https://doi.org/10.3138/9781442673946.

Hier, Sean P., and Joshua L. Greenberg. 2002. "Constructing a Discursive Crisis: Risk, Problematization, and Illegal Chinese in Canada." *Ethnic and Racial Studies* 25, no. 3: 490–513. https://doi.org/10.1080/01419870020036701.

HIV Justice Network. 2023. *Countries – Canada*. Last modified November 2023; accessed July 12, 2023. https://www.hivjustice.net/country/ca/.

HIV Legal Network. 2020. *Media Reporting: HIV and the Criminal Law*. Toronto: HIV Legal Network. https://www.hivlegalnetwork.ca/site/media-reporting-hiv-and-the-criminal-law/?lang=en.

– 2021. *HIV Criminalization, Women, and Gender-Diverse People: At the Margins*. Toronto: HIV Legal Network. https://www.hivlegalnetwork.ca/site/hiv-criminalization-women-and-gender-diverse-people-at-the-margins/?lang=en.

Housfather, Anthony. 2019. *TheCriminalizationof HIV Non-Disclosure in Canada: Report of the Standing Committee on Justice and Human Rights*. Ottawa: House of Commons.

"How to Have Sex in a Police State: One Approach." n.d. Accessed 19 November 2019. https://howtohavesexinapolicestate.tumblr.com/.

Hughes, Caitlin Elizabeth, Kari Lancaster, and Bridget Spicer. 2011. "How Do Australian News Media Depict Illicit Drug Issues? An Analysis of Print Media Reporting Across and Between Illicit Drugs, 2003–2008." *International Journal of Drug Policy* 22, no. 4 (July): 285–91. https://doi.org/10.1016/j.drugpo.2011.05.008.

Hunt, Julia. 2017. "'Fake News' Named Collin Dictionary's Word of the Year for 2017." *Independent*, 2 November. https://www.independent.co.uk/news/uk/home-news/fake-news-word-of-the-year-2017-collins-dictionary-donald-trump-kellyanne-conway-antifa-corbynmania-gender-fluidity-fidget-spinner-a8032751.html.

Infotendcias Group. 2012. "Media Convergence." In *The Handbook of Global Online Journalism*, edited by Eugenia Siapera and Andreas Veglis, 21–38. London: Wiley-Blackwell. https://doi.org/10.1002/9781118313978.

Jenkins, Henry. 2006. *Convergence Culture: Where Old and New Media Collide.* New York: New York University Press.

Jiwani, Yasmin. 2006. *Discourses of Denial: Meditations of Race, Gender, and Violence.* Vancouver: UBC Press. https://doi.org/10.59962/9780774855228.

Jiwani, Yasmin, and Mary Lynn Young. 2006. "Missing and Murdered Women: Reproducing Marginality in News Discourse." *Canadian Journal of Communication* 31, no. 4 (December): 895–917. https://doi.org/10.22230/cjc.2006v31n4a1825.

Jones, Tom. 2020. "The News Cycle of 2020: 'We're Drinking Out of a Fire Hose Every Night'." *Poynter*, 18 November. https://www.poynter.org/newsletters/2020/the-news-cycle-of-2020-were-drinking-out-of-a-fire-hose-every-night/.

Karlsson, Michael. 2011. "The Immediacy of Online News, the Visibility of Journalistic Processes and a Restructuring of Journalistic Authority." *Journalism* 12, no. 3 (April): 279–95. https://doi.org/10.1177/1464884910388223.

Keogh, Declan. 2017. "HIV Is Not a Crime." *NOW Magazine*, 12 January. https://nowtoronto.com/news/hiv-is-not-a-crime/.

Keung, Nicholas. 2016. "Media Accused of Racism in Reporting HIV-Related Crime." *Toronto Star*, 1 December. https://www.thestar.com/news/immigration/media-accused-of-racism-in-reporting-hiv-related-crime/article_3c48ddfd-8e6c-5476-a5d5-bf58b266f26d.html.

Khan, Ummni. 2014. "The Politics of Representation." In *Criminalizaiton, Representation, Regulation: Thinking Differently About Crime*, edited by Deborah Brock, Amanda Glasbeek, and Carmela Murdocca, 49–74. Toronto: University of Toronto Press.

Kilty, Jennifer M. 2021. "The Emotional Storying of Charles Ssenyonga as an HIV Sexual Predator in June Callwood's Trial Without End: A Shocking Story of Women and AIDS." In *Research Handbook on Law and Emotion*, edited by Susan A. Bandes, Jody Lynée Madeira, Kathryn D. Temple, and Emily Kidd White, 342–57. Cheltenham, UK: Elgar.

Kilty, Jennifer M., and Katarina Bogosavljevic. 2019. "Emotional Storytelling: Sensational Media and the Creation of the HIV Sexual Predator." *Crime, Media, Culture: An International Journal* 15 (April): 279–99. https://doi.org/10.1177/1741659018773813.

Kinsman, Gary. 2018. "AIDS Activism: Remembering Resistance Versus Socially Organized Forgetting." In *Seeing Red: HIV/AIDS and Public Policy in Canada*, edited by Suzanne Hindmarch, Michael Orsini, and Marilou Gagnon, 311–34. Toronto: University of Toronto Press. https://doi.org/10.3138/9781487510305-017.

Kirkup, Kyle. 2014–15. "Releasing Stigma: Police, Journalists and Crimes of HIV Non-Disclosure." *Ottawa Law Review* 46, no. 1: 127–60. http://doi.org/10.2139/ssrn.2503261.

Klinenberg, Eric. 2005. "Convergence: News Production in a Digital Age." *Annals of the American Academy of Political and Social Science* 597, no. 1 (January): 48–64.

Kolodzy, Janet. 2006. *Convergence Journalism: Writing and Reporting Across the News Media*. Oxford: Rowman and Littlefield.

Koskela, Merja. 2010. "From Bureaucrats to the Public on the Internet. Methodological Aspects of Intertextual Analysis." *Fachsprache* 32, nos. 1–2 (May): 54–63. https://doi.org/10.24989/fs.v32i1-2.1407.

Krieger, Nancy, Jarvis T. Chen, Pamela D. Waterman, Mathew V. Kiang, and Justin Feldman. 2015. "Police Killings and Police Deaths Are Public Health Data and Can Be Counted." *PLOS Medicine* 12, no. 12 (8 December): e1001915. https://doi.org/10.1371/journal.pmed.1001915.

Latour, Bruno. 1986. "Visualization and Cognition: Thinking with Eyes and Hands." *Knowledge and Society: Studies in the Sociology of Culture, Past and Present* 6: 1–40.

– 1987. *Science in Action*. Milton Keynes, UK: Open University Press.Latour, Bruno, and Steve Woolgar. 1986. *Laboratory Life: The Construction of Scientific Facts*. Princeton, NJ: Princeton University Press.

Lawson, Erica. 2014. "Disenfranchised Gried and Social Inequality: Bereaved African Canadians and Oppositional Narratives about Violent Deaths and Family Members." *Ethnic and Racial Studies* 37, no. 11 (September): 2092–109. https://doi.org/10.1080/01419870.2013.800569.

Lawson-Borders, Gracie. 2003. "Integrating New Media and Old Media: Seven Observations of Convergence as a Strategy for Best Practices in Media Organizations." *International Journal on Media Management* 5, no. 2: 91–9. https://doi.org/10.1080/14241270309390023.

Lester, Elli. 1992. "The AIDS Story and Moral Panic: How the Euro-African Press Constructs AIDS." *Howard Journal of Communications* 3, nos. 3–4 (January): 230–41. https://doi.org/10.1080/10646179209359752.

Levy, David A.L., and Rasmus Kleis Nielsen, eds. 2010. *The Changing Business of Journalism and Its Implications for Democracy*. Oxford: Reuters Institute for the Study of Journalism, University of Oxford.

Lewis, Justin, Andrew Williams, and Bob Franklin. 2008. "A Compromised Fourth Estate?" *Journalism Studies* 9, no. 1 (February): 1–20. https://doi.org/10.1080/14616700701767974.

Linell, Per. 1998. "Discourse across Boundaries: On Recontextualizations and the Blending of Voices in Professional Discourse." *Text* 18, no. 2 (April): 143–57. https://doi.org/10.1515/text.1.1998.18.2.143.

Lopez, William D. 2019. *Separated: Family and Community in the Aftermath of an Immigration Raid*. Baltimore, MD: Johns Hopkins University Press.

Loutfy, Mona, Mark Tyndall, Jean-Guy Baril, Julio S.G. Montaner, Rupert Kaul, and Catherine Hankins. 2014. "Canadian Consensus Statement on HIV and Its Transmission in the Context of Criminal Law." *Canadian Journal of Infectious Diseases and Medical Microbiology* 25, no. 3 (May/June): 135–40. https://doi.org/10.1155/2014/498459.

Lupton, Deborah. 1994. *Moral Threats and Dangerous Desires: AIDS in the News Media*. London: Taylor & Francis.

– 1999. *Risk*. New York: Taylor & Francis.

Magin, Melanie, and Peter Maurer. 2019. "Beat Journalism and Reporting." In *Oxford Research Encyclopedia of Communication*. Oxford: Oxford University Press. https://doi.org/10.1093/acrefore/9780190228613.013.905.

Marwick, Alice, and Rebecca Lewis. 2017. *Media Manipulation and Disinformation Online*. New York: Data & Society Research Institute.

Mawby, Rob C. 1999. "Visibility, Transparency and Police Media Relations." *Policing and Society* 9, no. 3 (July): 263–86. https://doi.org/10.1080/10439463.1999.9964816.

– 2010. "Police Corporate Communications, Crime Reporting, and the Shaping of Policing News." *Policing and Society* 20, no. 1 (March): 124–39. https://doi.org/10.1030/10439461003611526.

May, Katie. 2017. "Guilty Verdict Upheld in HIV Sexual Assault." *Winnipeg Free Press*, 7 July, 6.

Maynard, Robyn. 2017. *Policing Black Lives: State Violence in Canada from Slavery to the Present*. Halifax: Fernwood.

McClelland, Alexander. 2013. "Research at the Medico-Legal Borderland: Perspectives on HIV and Criminal Law." *Somatosphere*, 14 October. https://somatosphere.com/2013/research-at-the-medico-legal-borderland.html/.

– 2019a. "'Lock This Whore Up': Legal Violence and Flows of Information Precipitating Personal Violence Against People Criminalised for HIV-Related Crimes in Canada." *European Journal of Risk Regulation* 10, no. 1 (March): 132–47. https://doi.org/10.1017/err.2019.20.

– 2019b. *The Criminalization of HIV Non-Disclosure in Canada: Experiences of People Living with HIV*. n.p.: n.p. https://toolkit.hivjusticeworldwide.org/wp-content/uploads/2019/12/McClelland-Criminalization-2.pdf.

McCoy, Liza. 2006. "Keeping the Institution in View: Working with Interview Accounts of Everyday Experience." In *Institutional Ethnography as Practice*, edited by Dorothy E. Smith, 109–24. Lanham, MD: Rowman and Littlefield.

McGinty, Emma E., Alene Kennedy-Hendricks, Julia Baller, Jeff Niederdeppe, Sarah Gollust, and Colleen L. Barry. 2016. "Criminal Activity or Treatable Health Condition? News Framing of Opioid Analgesic Abuse in the United States, 1998–2013." *Psychiatric Services* 67, no. 4 (April): 405–12. https://doi.org/10.1176/appi.ps.201500065.

McIntyre, Mike. 2014a. "Conviction for Infecting Man with HIV." *Winnipeg Free Press*, 19 December, A5.

– 2014b. "Crown Closes Case in HIV Sex Assault Trial; Final Arguments to Begin." *Winnipeg Free Press*, 16 December. https://www.winnipegfreepress.com/breakingnews/2014/12/16/crown-closes-case-in-hiv-sex-assault-trial-final-arguments-to-begin.

– 2014c. "Lawyer Grills Male Accuser as HIV-Transmission Trial Begins." *Winnipeg Free Press*, 10 December, B2.

McKay, Fiona H., Samantha L. Thomas, Kate Holland, R. Warwick Blood, and Susan Kneebone. 2011. "'AIDS Assassins': Australian Media's Portrayal of HIV-Positive Refugees Who Deliberately Infect Others." *Journal of Immigrant and Refugee Studies* 9, no. 1 (February): 20–37. https://doi.org/10.1080/15562948.2011.547824.

McManus, John H. 2008. "The Commercialization of News." In *The Handbook of Journalism Studies*, edited by Karin Wahl-Jorgensen and Thomas Hanitzsch, 218–33. New York: Routledge.

– 2019. "Commodification of News." *International Encyclopedia of Journalism Studies*. https://doi.org/10.1002/9781118841570.iejs0063.

Menke, Manuel, Susanne Kinnebrock, Sonja Kretzschmar, Ingrid Aichberger, Marcel Broersma, Roman Hummel, Susanne Kirchhoff, Dimitri Prandner, Nelson Ribeiro, and Ramón Salaverría. 2019. "Insights from a Comparative Study into Convergence Culture in European Newsrooms." *Journalism Practice* 13, no. 8 (September): 946–50. https://doi.org/10.1080/17512786.2019.1642133.

Miller, David, and Kevin Williams. 1993. "Negotiating HIV/AIDS Information: Agendas, Media Strategies and the News." In *Getting the Message: News, Truth, and Power*, edited by John Eldridge, 126–42. Abingdon, UK: Routledge. https://doi.org/10.4324/9780203397404_chapter_6.

Miller, James. 2005. "African Immigrant Damnation Syndrome: The Case of Charles Ssenyonga." *Sexuality Research and Social Policy* 2, no. 2 (June): 31–50.

Miller, Peter, and Nikolas Rose. 1990. "Governing Economic Life." *Economy and Society* 19, no. 1 (February): 1–31. https://doi.org/10.1080/03085149000000001.

Mitchelstein, Eugenia, and Pablo J. Boczkowski. 2009. "Between Tradition and Change: A Review of Recent Research on Online New Production." *Journalism* 10, no. 5 (October): 562–86. https://doi.org/10.1177/1464884909106533.

Monahan, Torin, and Rodolfo D. Torres. 2010. *Schools Under Surveillance: Cultures of Control in Public Education*. New Brunswick, NJ: Rutgers University Press.

Monson, Sarah. 2017. "Ebola as African: American Media Discourses of Panic and Otherization." *Africa Today* 63, no. 3 (Spring): 3–27.

Motschall, Melissa, and Liqun Cao. 2002. "An Analysis of the Public Relations Role of the Police Public Relations Officer." *Police Quarterly* 5, no. 2 (June): 152–80. https://doi.org/10.1177/109861102129198084.

Moussa, Mario, and Ron Scapp. 1996. "The Practical Theorizing of Michel Foucault: Politics and Counter-Discourse." *Cultural Critique* 33 (Spring): 87–112. https://doi.org/10.2307/1354388.

Müller, Martin. 2015. "Assemblages and Actor-Networks: Rethinking Socio-Material Power, Politics and Space." *Geography Compass* 9, no. 1 (January): 27–41. https://doi.org/10.1111/gec3.12192.

Murdocca, Carmela. 2003. "When Ebola Came to Canada: Race and the Making of the Respectable Body." *Atlantis* 27, no. 2 (April): 24–31.

Mykhalovskiy, Eric. 2003. "Evidence-Based Medicine: Ambivalent Reading and the Clinical Recontextualization of Science." *Health: An Interdisciplinary Journal for the Social Study of Health, Illness, and Medicine* 7, no. 3 (July): 331–52. https://doi.org/10.1177/1363459303007003005.

– 2011. "The Problem of 'Significant Risk': Exploring the Public Health Impact of Criminalizing HIV Non-Disclosure." *Social Science and Medicine* 73, no. 5 (September): 668–75. https://doi.org/10.1016/j.socscimed.2011.06.051.

Mykhalovskiy, Eric, Colin Hastings, Leigha Comer, Julia Gruson-Wood, and Matthew Strang. 2021a. "Teaching Institutional Ethnography as an Alternative Sociology." In *The Palgrave Handbook of Institutional Ethnography*, edited by Paul C. Luken and Suzanne Vaughan, 47–65. Cham, Switzerland: Palgrave Macmillan. https://doi.org/10.1007/978-3-030-54222-1_4.

Mykhalovskiy, Eric, Colin Hastings, Chris Sanders, Michelle Hayman, and Laura Bisaillon. 2016. *"Callous, Cold and Deliberately Duplicitous": Racialization, Immigration and the Representation of HIV Criminalization in Canadian Mainstream Newspapers*. Toronto: n.p.

Mykhalovskiy, Eric, and Liza McCoy. 2002. "Troubling Ruling Discourses of Health: Using Institutional Ethnography in Community-Based Research." *Critical Public Health* 12, no. 1 (March): 17–37. https://doi.org/10.1080/09581590110113286.

Mykhalovskiy, Eric, Chris Sanders, Colin Hastings, and Laura Bisaillon. 2021b. "Explicitly Racialised and Extraordinarily Over-Represented: Black Immigrant Men in 25 Years of News Reports on HIV Non-Disclosure Criminal Cases in Canada." *Culture, Health & Sexuality* 23, no. 6 (June): 788–803. https://doi.org/10.1080/13691058.2020.1733095.

Namaste, Viviane. 2006. "Changes of Name and Sex for Transsexuals in Quebec: Understanding the Arbitrary Nature of Institutions." In *Sociology for Changing the World: Social Movements/Social Research*, edited by Caelie Frampton, Gary Kinsman, A.K. Thompson, and Kate Tilleczek, 160–73. Halifax: Fernwood.

Napoli, Philip M. 2010. *Audience Evolution: New Technologies and the Transformation of Media Audiences*. New York: Columbia University Press.

Nix, Justin, and Justin T. Pickett. 2017. "Third-Person Perceptions, Hostile Media Effects, and Policing: Developing a Theoretical Framework for

Assessing the Ferguson Effect." *Journal of Criminal Justice* 51 (July): 24–33. https://doi.org/10.1016/j.jcrimjus.2017.05.016.

Nylund, Mats. 2011. "The News-Generating Machine." *Journalism Practice* 5, no. 4 (August): 478–91. https://doi.org/10.1080/17512786.2011.575689.

O'Byrne, Patrick. 2011. "The Potential Public Health Effects of a Police Announcement About HIV Nondisclosure: A Case Scenario Analysis." *Policy, Politics & Nursing Practice* 12, no. 1 (February): 55–63. https://doi.org/10.1177/1527154411411484.

Oliver, Mary Beth. 2003. "African American Men as 'Criminal and Dangerous:' Implications of Media Portrayals of Crime on 'Criminalization' of African American Men." *Journal of African American Studies* 7, no. 2 (September): 3–18.

Parker, Richard, and Peter Aggleton. 2003. "HIV and AIDS-Related Stigma and Discrimination: A Conceptual Framework and Implications for Action." *Social Science and Medicine* 57, no. 1 (July): 13–24. https://doi.org/10.1016/s0277-9536(02)00304-0.

Parks, Lisa, and Nicole Starosielski, eds. 2015. *Signal Traffic: Critical Studies of Media Infrastructure*. Chicago: University of Illinois Press. https://doi.org/10.5406/illinois/9780252039362.001.0001.

Paterson, Chris. 2008. "What Is Ethnography?" In *Making News Online: The Ethnography of New Media Production*, Digital Formation, edited by Chris Paterson and David Domingo, 1–15. New York: Peter Lang.

Patton, Cindy. 1986. *Sex & Germs: The Politics of AIDS*. Montreal: Black Rose Books.

– 2005. "Outlaw Territory: Criminality, Neighborhoods, and the Edward Savitz Case." *Sexuality Research and Social Policy* 2, no. 2 (June): 63–75. https://doi.org/10.1525/srsp.2005.2.2.63.

Pavlik, John V. 2001. *Journalism and the New Media*. New York: Columbia University Press. https://doi.org/10.7312/pavl11482.

Persson, Asha, and Christy Newman. 2008. "Making Monsters: Heterosexuality, Crime, and Race in Recent Western Media Coverage of HIV." *Sociology of Health & Illness* 30, no. 4 (May): 632–46. https://doi.org/10.1111/j.1467-9566.2008.01082.x.

Petre, Caitlin. 2015. *The Traffic Factories: Metrics at Chartbeat, Gawker Media, and the New York Times*. New York: Tow Center for Digital Journalism.

– 2021. *All the News That's Fit to Click*. Princeton, NJ: Princeton University Press. https://doi.org/10.2307/j.ctv1htpf51.

Petty, Mary S. 2005. "Social Responses to HIV: Fearing the Outlaw." *Sexuality Research and Social Policy* 2, no. 2 (June): 76–88. https://doi.org/10.1525/srsp.2005.2.2.76.

Phillips, Angela. 2014. *Journalism in Context:Practiceand Theory for the Digital Age*. London: Routledge. https://doi.org/10.4324/9780203111741.

Picard, André. 2018. "Countries, Including Canada, Are Prosecuting People with HIV Because They Misunderstand Science, Leading Researchers Say." *Globe and Mail*, 27 July. https://www.theglobeandmail.com/canada/article -countries-including-canada-are-prosecuting-people-with-hiv-because/.

Plantin, Jean-Christophe, and Aswin Punathambekar. 2019. "Digital Media Infrastructures: Pipes, Platforms, and Politics." *Media Culture & Society* 41, no. 2 (March): 163–74. https://doi.org/10.1177/0163443718818376.

Poovey, Mary. 1998. *The History of the Modern Fact*. Chicago: University of Chicago Press.

Porter, Theodore M. 1995. *Trust in Numbers: The Pursuit of Objectivity in Science and Public Life*. Princeton, NJ: Princeton University Press. https://doi.org /10.1515/9730691210544.

Pough, Gwendolyn D. 2004. *CheckIt While I Wreck It: Black Womanhood, Hip-Hop Culture and the Public Sphere*. Boston: Northwestern University Press.

Quandt, T. 2008. "News Tuning and Content Management: An Observation Study of Old and New Routines in German Online Newsrooms." In *Making News Online: The Ethnography of New Media Production*, Digital Formation, edited by Chris Paterson and David Domingo, 77–97. New York: Peter Lang.

Quinn, Stephen. 2004. "An Intersection of Ideals: Journalism, Profits, Technology and Convergence." *Convergence* 10, no. 4 (December): 109–23.

Ramsey, Nancy. 2018. "Headline Stress Disorder: When Breaking News Is Bad for Your Health." *healthline*, 30 July 2018, archived 28 May 2023, at the Wayback Machine. https://web.archive.org/web/20230528105154 /https://www.healthline.com/health-news/headline-stress-disorder-when -breaking-news-is-bad-for-health.

Reeves, Joshua, and Jeremy Packer. 2013. "Police Media: The Governance of Territory, Speed, and Communication." *Communication and Critical/Cultural Studies* 10, no. 4 (December): 359–84. https://doi.org/10.1080/14791420.2013 .835053.

Reinardy, Scott. 2011. "Newspaper Journalism in Crisis: Burnout on the Rise, Eroding Young Journalists' Career Commitment." *Journalism* 12, no. 1 (January): 33–50. https://doi.org/10.1177/1464884910385188.

Reitmanova, Sylvia. 2009. "'Disease-Breeders' Among Us: Deconstructing Race and Ethnicity as Risk Factors of Immigrant Ill Health." *Journal of Medical Humanities* 30, no. 3 (September): 183–90. https://doi.org/10.1007 /s10912-009-9084-6.

Richardson, Linda. 2018. "HIV-Positive Man Going to Penitentiary for Aggravated Sex Assaults." Soo Today, 20 November. https://www.sootoday .com/local-news/hiv-positive-man-going-to-penitentiary-for-aggravated -sex-assaults-1128991.

Ritchie, Kevin. 2017. "Laws Criminalizing HIV Are Putting Vulnerable Women at Greater Risk." *NOW Magazine*, 11 January. https://nowtoronto

.com/news/laws-criminalizing-hiv-are-putting-vulnerable-women-at
-greater-risk/.

Rodriguez-Cayro, Kyli. 2018. "What Is Headline Stress Disorder? Here's How
to Protect Yourself from Anxiety About the News Cycle." *Bustle*, 28 June.
https://www.bustle.com/p/what-is-headline-stress-disorder-heres-how
-to-protect-yourself-from-anxiety-about-the-news-cycle-9611772.

Rose, Nikolas. 1988. "Calculable Minds and Manageable Individuals." *History
of the Human Sciences* 1 (October): 179–200.

Roth, Jenny, and Chris Sanders. 2018. "'Incorrigible Slag,' the Case of Jennifer
Murphy's HIV Non-Disclosure: Gender Norm Policing and the Production
of Gender-Class-Race Categories in Canadian News Coverage." *Women's
Studies International Forum* 68 (May–June): 113–20. https://doi.org
/10.1016/j.wsif.2018.03.004.

Ryan, Charlotte, Kevin M. Carragee, and William Meinhofer. 2001. "Theory
into Practice: Framing, the News Media, and Collective Action." *Journal of
Broadcasting and Electronic Media* 45, no. 1 (March): 175–82. https://
doi.org/10.1207/s15506878jobem4501_11.

Ryfe, David M. 2012. *Can Journalism Survive? An Inside Look in American
Newsrooms*. Malden, MA: Polity Press.

Sanders, Chris. 2014. "Discussing the Limits of Confidentiality: The Impact
of Criminalizing HIV Nondisclosure on Public Health Nurses' Counseling
Practices." *Public Health Ethics* 7, no. 3 (November): 253–60. https://
doi.org/10.1093/phe/phu032.

– 2015. "Examining Public Health Nurses' Documentary Practices: The
Impact of Criminalizing HIV Non-Disclosure on Inscription Styles." *Critical
Public Health* 25, no. 4 (August): 398–409. https://doi.org/10.1080/09581596
.2015.1019834.

Saridou, Theodora, Spyridou Lia-Paschalia, and Andreas Veglis. 2017.
"Churnalism on the Rise? Assessing Convergence Effects on Editorial
Practices." *Digital Journalism* 5, no. 8 (September): 1006–24. https://doi.org
/10.1080/21670811.2017.1342209.

Seale, Clove. 2003. "Health and Media: An Overview." *Sociology of Health &
Illness* 25: 513–31. https://doi.org/10.1111/1467-9566.t01-1-00356.

SERO Project. n.d. *HIV Is Not a Crime National Training Academy*. Accessed 31
July 2023. https://www.seroproject.com/hinac/.

Sewell, Abigail A., and Kevin A. Jefferson. 2016. "Collateral Damage: The
Health Effects of Invasive Police Encounters in New York City." *Journal of
Urban Health* 93, no. S1 (April): 42–67. https://doi.org/10.1007/s11524-015
-0016-7.

Shoemaker, Pamela J. 2001. "Review of Radical Media: Rebellious
Communication and Social Movements, by John D.H. Downing, with
Tamara Villarreal Ford, Genéve Gil, and Laura Stein." *Journalism and Mass*

Communications Quarterly 78, no. 3 (September): 617–18. https://doi.org
/10.1177/107769900107300311.

Smith, Dorothy E. 1987. *The Everyday World as Problematic: A Feminist Sociology.*
Toronto: University of Toronto Press.

– 1990. *The Conceptual Practices of Power.* Boston: Northeastern University Press.

– 1993. *Texts, Facts, and Femininity: Exploring the Relations of Ruling.* London:
Routledge. https://doi.org/10.2307/2074806.

– 2001. "Texts and the Ontology of Organizations and Institutions." *Studies in
Culture, Organizations, and Societies* 7, no. 2: 159–98. https://doi.org
/10.1080/10245280108523557.

– 2002. "Institutional Ethnography." In *Qualitative Research in Action,*
edited by Tim May, 17–52. London: Sage. https://doi.org/10.4135
/9781849209656.

– 2005. *Institutional Ethnography: A Sociology for People.* Oxford: AlraMira Press.

Smith, George W. 1990. "Political Activist as Ethnographer." *Social Problems* 37,
no. 4 (November): 629–48. https://doi.org/10.2307/800586.

Smith, Joanna 2016. "Advocates Hopeful Canada Will Stop Criminalizing
Non-Disclosure of HIV Status." *Victoria Times Colonist*, 29 December, D1.

Solin, Anna. 2004. "Intertextuality as Mediation: On the Analysis of Intertextual
Relations in Public Discourse." *Text* 24, no. 2 (June): 267–96. https://doi
.org/10.1515/text.2004.010.

Sontag, Susan. 1989. *AIDS and Its Metaphors.* New York: Farrar, Straus, and Giroux.

Spector, Nicole. 2017. "Headline Stress Disorder: How to Cope with the
Anxiety Caused by the 24/7 News Cycle." *NBC News*, 16 December.
https://www.nbcnews.com/better/health/what-headline-stress-disorder
-do-you-have-it-ncna830141.

Spolum, Maren M., William D. Lopez, Daphne C. Watkins, and Paul J.
Fleming. 2023. "Police Violence: Reducing the Harms of Policing through
Public Health-Informed Alternative Response Programs." *American Journal
of Public Health* 113, no. S1 (January): S37–S42. https://doi.org/10.2105
/AJPH.2022.307107.

Steense, Steen, and Laura Ahva. 2015. "Theories of Journalism in a Digital
Age: An Exploration and Introduction." *Digital Journalism* 3, no. 1 (January):
1–18.

Stosny, Steven. 2017. "Overcoming Headline Stress Disorder." *Psychology
Today*, 4 March. https://www.psychologytoday.com/us/blog/anger-in
-the-age-entitlement/201703/overcoming-headline-stress-disorder.

Surette, Ray. 1998. *Media, Crime, and Criminal Justice: Images and Realities.*
Belmont, CA: Wadsworth.

Surette, Ray, and Alfredo Richard. 1995. "Public Information Officers: A
Descriptive Study of Crime News Gatekeeper." *Journal of Criminal Justice* 23,
no. 4: 325–36. https://doi.org/10.1016/0047-2352(95)00023-J.

Taylor, Stuart. 2008. "Outside the Outsiders: Media Representations of Drug Use." *Probation Journal* 55, no. 4 (December): 369–87. https://doi.org/10.1177/0264550508096493.

Theriot, Matthew T. 2009. "School Resource Officers and the Criminalization of Student Behavior." *Journal of Criminal Justice* 37, no. 3 (May–June): 280–7. https://doi.org/10.1016/j.jcrimjus.2009.04.008.

Timmermans, Stefan, and Jonathan Gabe. 2002. "Introduction: Connecting Criminology and Sociology of Health and Illness." *Sociology of Health & Illness* 24, no. 5 (September): 501–16. http://doi.wiley.com/10.1111/1467-9566.00306.

Trussler, Terry, and Rick Marchand. 2005. "HIV/AIDS Community-Based Research." *New Directions for Adult and Continuing Education* 2005, no. 105 (Spring): 43–54. http://doi.wiley.com/10.1002/ace.168.

Tsfati, Yariv, and Yoram Peri. 2006. "Mainstream Media Skepticism and Exposure to Sectorial and Extranational News Media: The Case of Israel." *Mass Communication & Society* 9, no. 2 (May): 165–87. https://doi.org/10.1207/s15327825mcs0902_3.

Tuchman, Gaye. 1978. *Making News: A Study of the Social Construction of Reality.* New York: Free Press.

Tumber, Howard. 1999. "Introduction." In *News: A Reader*, edited by Howard Tumber, xv–xix. Oxford: Oxford University Press.

Turner, James. 2013. "No Preliminary Hearing for Woman Accused of Giving HIV to Partner." *Winnipeg Free Press*, 15 September. https://www.winnipegfreepress.com/breakingnews/2013/09/15/no-preliminary-hearing-for-woman-accused-of-giving-hiv-to-partner.

– 2014. "Woman Loses Fight to Ditch Her HIV Charge." *Winnipeg Free Press*, 4 April, A4.

– 2017. "Woman Convicted of Sexual Assault in HIV-Disclosure Case Appeals to Supreme Court." *CBC News*, 30 July. https://www.cbc.ca/news/canada/manitoba/schenkels-hiv-appeal-supreme-court-1.4228041.

Turow, Joseph. 1997. *Breaking up America: Advertisers and the New Media World.* Chicago: University of Chicago Press. https://doi.org/10.7208/chicago/9780226817514.001.0001.

Usher, Nikki. 2014. *Making News at the New York Times.* Ann Arbor: University of Michigan Press. https://doi.org/10.2307/j.ctv65sxjj.

– 2018. "Breaking News Production Processes in US Metropolitan Newspapers: Immediacy and Journalistic Authority." *Journalism* 19, no. 1 (January): 21–36. https://doi.org/10.1177/1464884916689151.

van Dijck, José, Thomas Poell, and Martijn de Wall. 2018. *The Platform Society: Public Values in a Connective World.* New York: Oxford University Press.

van Dijk, Teun A. 1988. *News as Discourse.* Hillsdale, NJ: Lawrence Erlbaum.

– 2018. "Discourse and Migration." In *Qualitative Research in European Migration Studies*, edited by Ricard Zapata-Barrero and Evren Yalaz, 227–54. Cham, Switzerland: Springer.

Van Leuven, Sarah, Bart Vanhaelewyn, and Karin Raeymaeckers. 2021. "From One Division of Labor to the Other: The Relation between Beat Reporting, Freelancing, and Journalistic Autonomy." *Journalism Practice* 15, no. 9 (October): 1203–21. https://doi.org/10.1080/17512786.2021.1910982.

Vu, Hong Tien. 2014. "The Online Audience as Gatekeeper: The Influence of Reader Metrics on News Editorial Selection." *Journalism* 15, no. 8 (November): 1094–110. https://doi.org/10.1177/1464884913504259.

Watney, Simon. 1987. *Policing Desire: Pornography, AIDS, and the Media.* Minneapolis: University of Minnesota Press.

Weait, Matthew. 2007. *Intimacy and Responsibility: TheCriminalisationof HIV Transmission.* Abingdon, UK: Routledge-Cavendish. https://doi.org/10.4324/9780203937938.

Webster, Fiona, Kathleen Rice, and Abhimanyu Sud. 2020. "A Critical Content Analysis of Media Reporting on Opioids: The Social Construction of an Epidemic." *Social Science and Medicine* 244 (January): 112642. https://doi.org/10.1016/j.socscimed.2019.112642.

Wechsler, Steph. 2021. "A Year of Mapping Media Impacts of the Pandemic in Canada: COVID-19 Media Impact Map for Canada Update, March 11, 2021." *J Source: The Canadian Journalism Project*, 11 March. https://j-source.ca/a-year-of-mapping-media-impacts-of-the-pandemic-in-canada-covid-19-media-impact-map-for-canada-update-march-11-2021/.

Weir, Lorna, and Eric Mykhalovskiy. 2010. *Global Public Health Vigilance: Creating a World on Alert.* New York: Routledge.

Wente, Margaret. 2003. "Do the Right Thing: With HIV Rates Rising, Why Are Some of the Infected Condemning Their Partners to an Unnecessary Fate?" *Globe and Mail*, 29 November, A23.

White, David Manning. 1950. "The Gatekeeper." *Journalism Quarterly* 27, no. 4 (September): 383–90.

Wilson, Katelyn. 2022. "'I Do Not Infect Anyone,' Fighting for Change to End HIV Non-Disclosure Prosecution." *CTV News Barrie*, 2 February. https://barrie.ctvnews.ca/i-do-not-infect-anyone-fighting-for-change-to-end-hiv-non-disclosure-prosecution-1.5765502.

Winters, Maike, Anna Larsson, Jan Kowalski, and Carl Johan Sundberg. 2019. "The Association Between Quality Measures of Medical University Press Releases and Their Corresponding News Stories – Important Information Missing." *PLoS ONE* 14, no. 6 (June): e0217295. https://doi.org/10.1371/journal.pone.0217295.

Wood, Lesley J. 2014. *Crisis and Control: The Militarization of Protest Policing.* London: Pluto Press.

Zelizer, Barbie. 2017. *What Journalism Could Be.* Cambridge: Polity Press.

Zhang, Shixin Ivy. 2012. "The Newsroom of the Future: Newsroom Convergence Models in China." *JournalismPractice* 6, nos. 5–6 (October): 776–87. https://doi.org/10.1080/17512786.2012.667281.

Court Cases

R. v. Cuerrier, 1998 SCR 371.

Index

activating texts, phrase, 36, 36n1
activism, radical HIV, 4
activist interventions: creating
  texts for news production, 121–7;
  intervening in crime story reports,
  102–6; relational work, 127–34;
  as spokespeople in mainstream
  press, 106–16; text production
  work, 116–21
advocacy organizations, 66, 119, 147;
  media training, 141
advocates, intervening in media
  discourse, 141
African, Caribbean, and Black (ACB)
  communities, 23; criminal justice
  time and, 39; living with HIV and
  in Canada, 23–4; people living
  with HIV, 37–8, 122–3
African, Caribbean, and Black
  (ACB) people: HIV criminal cases
  involving, 130, 133–4; mainstream
  media and, 132; overrepresentation
  of, 23, 37, 123, 142
African and Caribbean Council on
  HIV/AIDS, Ontario, 23
Aggleton, Peter, 26
AIDS ACTION NEWS! (publication), 4
AIDS ACTION NOW!, 7; George
  Smith, 4

AIDS service organizations (ASOs),
  6, 23, 65, 101, 116, 138
Allain, Carol Ann, 4
American Medical Association, 95
American Public Health
  Association, 95
assemblage, definition of, 93–4

beat reporting, 30
BIPOC communities, 5, 97
Black activists, 4
"Black counter-discourse," 133
Black Lives Matter movement, 89
Blatchford, Christie, 38–40, 42
Broersma, Marcel, 84
Brown, Michael, 89
Bruser, David, 42
Butler-McPhee, Janet, 107; Legal
  Network (LN), 107, 107n2, 110–11,
  113, 116–17, 127–9

"Callous, Cold and Deliberately
  Duplicitous" (community report),
  37, 122
Callwood, June, 25
Canada: activism to resist and
  reform HIV criminalization
  in, 22–4; HIV non-disclosure,
  19–21

INSTITUTIONAL ETHNOGRAPHY: STUDIES IN THE SOCIAL ORGANIZATION OF KNOWLEDGE

Series Editor: Eric Mykhalovskiy, York University

Published to date:

Simply Institutional Ethnography: Creating a Sociology for People / Dorothy E. Smith and Alison I. Griffith (2022)